Momat Kitenge Felix

Natural delivery after previous caesarean section

Momat Kitenge Felix

Natural delivery after previous caesarean section

Development and validation of the PAUM predictive score

ScienciaScripts

Cover image: www.ingimage.com

This book is a translation from the original published under ISBN 978-620-2-54673-7.

Publisher:
Sciencia Scripts
is a trademark of
Dodo Books Indian Ocean Ltd. and OmniScriptum S.R.L publishing group

120 High Road, East Finchley, London, N2 9ED, United Kingdom
Str. Armeneasca 28/1, office 1, Chisinau MD-2012, Republic of Moldova, Europe
Printed at: see last page
ISBN: 978-620-8-31744-7

Table of contents:

Natural delivery after a previous Caesarean section: it's possible

Development and validation of the PAUM predictive score

By Félix Momat Kitenge

Dedication

To my Parents ;

To my loving Wife and worthy Mother, carrier of a thrice scarred uterus;

To my lovely children;

To all women with a scarred uterus;

I dedicate this book to you.

PREFACE

"Tota mulier in utero" (Hippocrates) *[The whole woman (is) in the womb*].

Here's a provocative maxim by the great Hippocrates of Cos, who could not have survived the opprobrium he would have attracted had he lived in the XXIe Century! This murderous phrase was perpetuated to satiety by all Enlightenment physicians after men had invaded the sacred domain of "*obstetrices*" in the XVIe century, those worthy heirs of the distant boarders of the College of Sais in ancient Egypt. This idea, which persisted explicitly until after the First World War, is still implicit today if we consider all the injustices suffered by women, because of their femininity, in most human societies.

Today, this aphorism may seem hypocritically shocking, but Hippocrates was merely the son of an era dominated by a societal machismo whose current followers are merely fighting a rearguard action doomed to failure. With the scene thus set, it's time for a happy rereading of our original sentence!

In fact, in his "Isagoge breves", published in 1954, Jacopo Berengario da Carpi, who produced the first accurate description of the uterus as we know it, described it as the only organ worthy of reproduction in his 1514 publication. In fact, unlike the father, the uterus is the organ that enables the woman and mother to be in biological communion, or better still, in permanent symbiosis with the future newborn and already "*homunculus*", throughout pregnancy, before being taken over by the mother's breasts from birth to weaning. It is therefore a noble and respectable organ in view of its purpose, which is to be both the natural receptacle for the beginning of life, its preservation and its passage to the world of the descendants *of Homo sapiens*!

What's more, it's common knowledge that most women have a natural desire to become mothers, a feeling shared by the majority of women.

African women. Particularly in Africa, women are distressed by the thought of not being able to carry a pregnancy, a situation fraught with social ostracism at the level of the extended family unit and the community as a whole. This brings back memories of the early years of my obstetric practice, when we were constantly confronted with the major complication of previous caesarean sections by corporal vertical incision: uterine rupture at the end of pregnancy, most often with a dead fetus. In most cases, the surgical solution was a subtotal interannexal hysterectomy, without anyone having the courage to inform the woman or her partner: *O tempora, O mores*! At the time, it was not unusual to see a former patient, accompanied by her entire family, demanding the return of her uterus after several months of amenorrhoea! Similarly, dilapidated and literally shattered uteruses were surgically repaired with the meticulousness of a watchmaker, in the hope of preserving patients' future maternity!

Of course, Caesarean section is no longer what it was after Jakob Nufer's feat in 1500: a veritable killing machine! Today, it's a surgical procedure that generally takes place in a safe environment when it's scheduled or performed under the best possible conditions, with healing proceeding impeccably afterwards. However, as with any other surgical procedure, complications can never be completely ruled out, especially in the case of an emergency C-section in a resource-constrained environment characterized by a lack of qualified healthcare personnel, infrastructure and appropriate equipment.

Obstetricians are faced with two attitudes, which are in fact the terms of two well-debated alternatives, in the presence of a scarred uterus due to a previous Caesarean section. Edwin Cragin's century-old opinion "*Once a Caesarean, always a Caesarean*" is no longer valid, for two reasons: prolonged labor lasting several days, high incidence of rickets and pelvic malformations, pre-syntocinon discovery period and dangerous surgical conditions; secondly, the fact that the C-section rate has over time proved to be below the cut-off point set for the risk of C-section among former Caesareans.

In view of the above, predictive models, within the framework of evidence-based medicine, have proved necessary to predict the risk of a failed vaginal delivery following a previous caesarean section. The author of the present thesis has thus continued in the same vein that very few before him had dared to tackle. What's more, he has done so boldly in a multicenter study, under very difficult environmental conditions and considering anamnestic and clinical parameters within the reach of any qualified health personnel, working in the peripheral maternity units of any health system in countries with limited resources in general, and those of sub-Saharan Africa in particular. This will have the triple merit of contributing to the reduction of maternal and perinatal morbidity and mortality by improving the quality of indications for vaginal delivery, increasing prophylactic caesarean section rates and better selecting patients for the therapeutic test. Ultimately, this is the type of scientific work that falls into the niche of research whose applicability requires no additional funding to effectively resolve a concrete problem facing the community.

Congratulations and thanks to the author!

Jean-Baptiste KAKOMA SAKATOLO ZAMBÈZE MD, MMed/OG, PhD, AESM

Professor Emeritus of Gynaecology-Obstetrics, Public Health & Parasitology

Honorary Rector of the University of Lubumbashi

INTRODUCTION

Pregnancy is a particular physiological state which, in the majority of cases, leads spontaneously to vaginal delivery. However, accidents of various kinds can disrupt its progress and compromise the fetal and/or maternal prognosis, thus constituting an indication for Caesarean section. Once intended solely for the treatment of major mechanical dystocies, Caesarean section surgery has now become an easy procedure, both in terms of the ease with which it can be performed and the lower morbidity and mortality for the mother-child couple.

The extraordinary progress made over the last four decades in surgical and anaesthetic techniques, the considerable revolution in the nursing service for fragile newborns, the post-operative patient monitoring service, and the development of pharmacology, have led to a significant diversification of indications and a marked increase in frequency.

Caesarean section rates have been rising in most countries over the past 20 years. This trend is increasingly exposing women to the situation of scarred uteri in future pregnancies. Currently, in industrialized countries, C-section rates are well above 15%, the threshold long defined as a maximum by the WHO. From 2010 to 2011, for example, the following rates were recorded: 20.8% in France; 24.7% in the USA; 24.9% in Spain; 26.6% in Canada and 42% in Mexico. The increase in caesarean section rates in the West has been accompanied by a proportional benefit for the mother-child couple.

Today, the maternal mortality ratio is less than 3 per 100,000 live births, and perinatal mortality is almost zero. The latest OECD report, including health indicators for 30 countries, shows caesarean section rates ranging from around 15% in the Netherlands, Finland and Iceland to over 40% in Mexico, Turkey, China and Brazil.

In developing countries, mainly in Sub-Saharan Africa, despite technological delays, Caesarean section rates are on the rise: in Lubumbashi (DRC), the frequency of Caesarean sections rose from 1.4% in 1995 to 1.97% in 1999 (an increase of 34%); in Senegal, the rate was 7.5% in 2000; in Niger, the C-section rate rose from 8.45% in 1992 to 13.56% in 2001, and in Congo Brazzaville from 2.4% in 1997 to 8.3% in 2002.

The direct consequence of this increase in caesarean section rates is an increase in the number of patients with scar uteri. At the end of the XXème century and the beginning of the XXIème century, the frequency of scar uteri varied from 6 to 12% in countries with a high level of health development. In France, between 1995 and 2010, the prevalence of scar uteri increased from 8 to 11%. In Australia, Appleton et al. reported, in a multicenter study, a rate of 9.2% of scar uteri in 2000 and 2003. Cassignol and Rudigoz confirmed that up to 10% of patients who gave birth had a scar uterus.

In countries with a low level of health development, as in Africa, the prevalence observed over the years varies from one country to another: the prevalence of deliveries on scarred uteri was 3% (1994), 6% (2000) in Morocco (Casablanca), according to Cassignol and Rudigoz; 7% in Cameroon (Yaoundé) and 7.7% in Tanzania (Dar-Es-Salam) in 2004, according to Zelop. The same author reports a rate of 9.2% in Rwanda (Kigali) in 2005. And 8.45% in the DRC (Kinshasa) in 2013, according to Boffendakini.

The health of mothers and children is inextricably linked, and the development of society as a whole depends to a large extent on their health. Since its creation in 1948, the WHO has focused much of its efforts on maternal and child health, defining key interventions for safe motherhood: good nutrition and health care for women from infancy, family planning integrated into primary health care, prenatal care and skilled attendance at birth, and access to essential obstetric care in emergencies.

Several factors have been identified to explain health disarray in developing countries: poverty, inadequate health services, their inaccessibility or, quite simply, their inadequate distribution throughout the country, as well as, in some cases, poor distribution of education and information. We also question certain ethno-cultural factors that promote early marriage and high rates of childbirth: traditional practices relating to gestation and childbirth, medical practices that are less reassuring for mothers and their newborns.

Caesarean section remains the main etiology of scar uteri in developing countries, particularly the DRC. Complications during pregnancy remain exceptional, and are represented by placental implantation anomalies (placenta previa, accreta, increta and percreta) and uterine rupture, a major complication most often occurring during labor. The treatment of scar uteri has been the subject of recommendations by learned obstetric societies, in view of the increasing incidence of scar uteri.

The widespread use of segmental caesarean sections and the progress made over the last two decades in managing the labour of patients with a scar uterus, thanks in particular to electronic labour monitoring, have contributed to a change in obstetrical behaviour, allowing VBACs to be performed with what is considered satisfactory safety, despite the fear of uterine rupture. The fear of uterine rupture and the absence of a codified, unanimous attitude to births with a scar uterus have led to a decrease in the rate of VBACs.

The choice of mode of delivery, in the case of a previous caesarean section, should take into account the assessment of potential maternal and neonatal complications of each delivery route. The recommendations issued by ACOG, SOGC and RCOG stress that uterine testing, which is a reasonable option, must take into account the place of delivery, its technical facilities, the characteristics of the patient, the qualifications of the nursing staff, obstetrical factors and obstetrical practices. However, VBAC and CPAC also entail risks for the mother-child couple.

In the case of a scarred uterus, vaginal delivery is acceptable only if there is a reduced risk of maternal-fetal morbidity and mortality. While the option of vaginal delivery is rarely discussed when the situation appears favorable (absence of recurrent cause of caesarean section, segmental scar), high-risk obstetrical situations (potentially recurrent indication for first caesarean section, undocumented previous caesarean section, multiple pregnancy, breech presentation, macrosomia, borderline pelvis, multiple scars) generally constitute a contraindication to uterine testing.

Today, the scar uterus is a risk factor for fetomaternal morbidity in subsequent pregnancies, irrespective of the route of delivery. This is due to the lack of unanimity among obstetric teams on the attitude to adopt to deliveries in a scar uterus.

The choice of mode of delivery, in the case of a previous caesarean section, should be based on a comparison of the maternal and neonatal complications of each route of delivery. However, neither uterine testing nor elective caesarean section is without risk for the mother-child pair.

The study of fetomaternal risk factors for UA is an important step in improving obstetric knowledge of the determinants of the UA route. Such a study should discuss, in our setting, the association between operative route, uterine test, uterine test failure and maternal-fetal morbidity and mortality, as obstetric practice decisions must take these different parameters into account.

There is, in fact, a correlation between uterine test failure and uterine rupture, with both being synergistic factors in morbidity and mortality for the mother-child pair. What's more, failure of the uterine test, if poorly managed, increases the risk of uterine rupture with fetal and/or maternal death.

The determinants of fetal-maternal outcome and uterine testing can be easily identified and should necessarily guide us in the choice of the route of delivery on scar uterus in order to contribute positively to the reduction of fetal-maternal morbidity related to this delivery.

To our knowledge, neither a predictive score nor determinants of fetomaternal outcome and uterine testing have yet been defined in the DRC. Few studies have highlighted the increased incidence of deliveries with scarred uteri. In 2013, at the Cliniques Universitaires de Kinshasa, the frequency was 8.45%, with maternal morbidity (uterine rupture) of 4.6%, zero maternal mortality and perinatal mortality of 29%, whereas thirty years earlier, at the same institution, the frequency was 2.43%, with maternal morbidity (uterine rupture) of 11.1%, maternal mortality of 0.69% and perinatal mortality of 90%. With a view to contributing to the prevention and/or minimization of the risk of maternal morbidity and mortality in cases of parturition on a scarred uterus in an obstetrical environment where the technical facilities and qualifications of nursing staff are sorely lacking, and to assessing the management of CUA, we conducted a multicenter study in four hospitals in three economically and socio-culturally different areas of the DRC (Kinshasa, Lubumbashi and Mbuji-Mayi).

While the provincial city of Kinshasa is the country's capital, with a highly heterogeneous population in political, social and economic terms, the city of Lubumbashi, capital of Haut-Katanga Province, is mainly a mining town, with an equally heterogeneous population, both socio-culturally and economically; while the city of Mbuji-Mayi, generally homogeneous, is mainly populated by ethnic Luba, whose socio-economic activities are less structured.

The principle of predicting the risk of delivery on a scarred uterus is defined as a clinical process that starts by combining the elements of the anamnesis, clinical and paraclinical examinations to establish a better fetomaternal prognosis for a given patient.

What then are the determinants of fetal-maternal outcome and uterine testing in gestational carriers of a scarred uterus?

Several hypotheses have been formulated, the three main ones being :

- the frequency of delivery on a scarred uterus is relatively high in our environment;
- Pregnancies in a scarred uterus are associated with high maternal and perinatal morbidity and mortality;
- well-organized uterine tests based on a predictive score could make a significant contribution to reducing and/or preventing morbidity and mortality in mother-child pairs.

The overall objective of the present study is to generate knowledge that contributes to the rational management of scar uterus deliveries in hospital settings, in a resource-limited environment.

Specifically, the study aims to :

- To determine the frequency of scar uterus deliveries in the DRC;
- Assessing maternal-fetal morbidity and mortality related to mode of delivery in scar uterus ;
- Identify factors associated with uterine test outcome;
- Develop a predictive score for the outcome of uterine testing.

This study is divided into four parts:

- The first part is a review of the literature on delivery in a scar uterus.
- The second part is a multicenter study of scar-uterine deliveries in the DRC. In addition to the methodology, this part successively presents the frequency of scar uterus deliveries, termination routes and maternal and perinatal morbidity and mortality, as well as the determinants of maternal-fetal outcome and uterine testing.
- The third concerns the development of a predictive score for the outcome of uterine testing, its indications, reliability and cost-

effectiveness.

- The final section is devoted to a general discussion of the results.
- A general conclusion and recommendations conclude this work.

PART ONE:
OVERVIEW OF BIRTHS ON SCAR UTERUS: A REVIEW OF THE LITERATURE LITERATURE
Chapter 1

1. Assessing the quality of the uterine scar

The decision to choose a delivery route in a scarred uterus is based on an assessment of the quality of the uterine scar, which requires a combination of anamnestic, clinical and para-clinical arguments.

1.1. Elements correlated with previous caesarean section

1.1.1. Type of hysterotomy

Of all uterine scars, corporal hysterotomies and T-incisions are considered to be the weakest and the most likely to cause uterine rupture. Several studies, including those by Pridjian and Papiernick, have corroborated this finding:

Pridjian [21] reported the frequency of uterine rupture according to the type of incision:

- *J* Low transverse incision: 0.2 to 0.8%.
- *J* Low longitudinal incision: 0.5 to 6.5%.
- *J* T-shaped incision: 4.3% to 8.8
- *J* Corporal incision: 4.3% to 8.8

Papiernick [22], in his series, notes even higher frequencies:

- *J* Strict corporal incision: 6 to 33%.
- *J* Segmental - corporal incision: 25% of incision

Thus, the consensus on the absolute contraindication of uterine testing for corporal and T-shaped incisions has been formally established.

1.1.2. Previous vaginal delivery

The notion of vaginal delivery, after caesarean section, has a good prognosis for the subsequent pregnancy, as intercalary delivery increases the chances of a successful uterine test in the subsequent pregnancy without increasing the risk of uterine rupture.

Cosson et al [23] compared the routes of delivery of two groups of patients with uni-cicatric uteri, some with a history of vaginal deliveries and others with no history of vaginal deliveries. In their study, they found that 21% of prophylactic caesareans and 79% of uterine tests were performed in the first group, compared with 50/50 parity in the second. In parturients with a history of natural vaginal deliveries, they found a 90% uterine test success rate and a 10% failure rate, resulting in 29.7% Caesarean sections and 70.3% vaginal deliveries, compared with 81% uterine test success rate and 19% failure rate, resulting in 59.4% vaginal deliveries and 40.6% vaginal deliveries in parturients with no history of vaginal deliveries.

Similarly, the notion of intercalary curettage is not a contraindication to uterine testing.

1.1.3. No indication for previous caesarean section

It is standard practice to perform scano-pelvimetry when the indication for a previous caesarean section is unknown, either immediately after the caesarean section or later in the subsequent pregnancy [24].

Scano-pelvimetry is performed to assess the size of the pelvis. According to the criteria evaluated by Magnin [25], this examination plays a very important role in deciding the mode of delivery for the next pregnancy. In the case of a shrunken pelvis, a prophylactic caesarean section is routinely performed, whereas in the case of a borderline pelvis, the decision depends essentially on the data obtained from the cephalo-pelvic confrontation, bearing in mind, however, that the ultrasound assessment of fetal weight is often erroneous.

Radiopelvimetry is not a good indicator for the mother, as it takes neither fetal volume nor presentation into account. Thus, a cephalo-pelvic comparison by ultrasound measurement of the fetal biparietal diameter combined with maternal radiopelvimetry remains an important element in the decision regarding the delivery route [25].

1.1.4. Length of labor before indication of first cesarean section

According to Papiernick [22], cervical dilatation greater than or equal to 4 cm at the time of Caesarean section appears to be a good prognostic factor for achieving vaginal delivery in subsequent pregnancies.

Demianczuk [26] found a 27% success rate for the uterine test in the group of patients with cervical dilatation of less than 3 cm at the time of the first caesarean section, compared with 69% in the group with cervical dilatation of 3 cm or more.

In his study, Lehmann [27] concludes that the longer the duration of labor, the higher the failure rate of the uterine test.

Ultimately, a prolonged first stage of labour with obvious stagnation of dilatation is often associated with a failed uterine test; and a caesarean section performed after a failed long labour with long ruptured membranes will result in a more fragile scar [28].

1.1.5. Postpartum Endometritis

In 2003, in his 12-year study, Shipp [29] showed a link between post-partum endometritis with a temperature > 38°C and the risk of uterine rupture during uterine testing. This risk is thought to be due to poor healing caused by bacterial infection.

Isolated fever during labor does not therefore appear to be a risk factor. Only proven post-partum endometritis may lead to contraindication of the vaginal route and prophylactic caesarean section, while any other febrile sequelae will only lead to closer monitoring of a uterine scar test in the next pregnancy [24].

I.2. Terrain-related elements

I.2.1 Age and parity of pregnant women

Pregnant women's age alone does not appear to be a factor influencing scar quality [30].

The association of "large multiparity" and "scar uterus" theoretically entails an increased risk of uterine rupture. In a study of 45 uterine tests in large multiparous women with scar uteruses, 27 parturients (61%) delivered vaginally, with 2 uterine ruptures (4.4%) and 2 scar dehiscences [31].

I.2.2 Multi-scar uterus

Most authors consider the multi-scar uterus to be an indication for iterative caesarean section [21]. According to A.C.O.G. recommendations [16], there is no contraindication to uterine testing on multi-scar uterus, provided that patients are carefully selected and optimally monitored.

In the 1980s, the presence of several uterine scars was considered a contraindication to uterine testing. Since then, the low morbidity of uterine testing on scarred uteri has reduced the number of contraindications. Some authors have even authorized uterine testing in parturients with multi-scar uteri [32, 33].

In Riyadh, Chattopadhay [34] performed 50% prophylactic caesarean sections and the same number of uterine tests on a total of 230 bi-scarred uteruses, resulting in 90% vaginal deliveries and 10% emergency caesarean sections, giving a total of 55.2% caesarean sections and 44.8% vaginal deliveries. These deliveries included one case of incomplete uterine rupture (0.8%) without alteration of maternal-fetal prognosis, one case of hysterectomy for uterine atony after caesarean section for failure of labour and macrosomia, and one maternal death from placenta previa in the prophylactic caesarean section group.

In conclusion, uterine testing on bi-cicatric uterus is a reasonable alternative.

1.2.3. Educational level and marital status

In a study carried out in Niger, Hamet et al [35] refer to a culturally diverse population of parturients and conclude that any difficulty in vaginal delivery is attributed to a problem of infidelity to the husband, and that only deliveries that become complicated in the village are reluctantly referred to health facilities.

For other authors, the level of education is an important element to take into account, because less educated women do not respect the prenatal consultation schedule and do not observe any discipline in the delivery room [36].

1.3. Factors related to the current pregnancy

1.3.1. Intergenic interval

Several studies show an increased rate of uterine rupture in the case of closely spaced pregnancies.

A minimum interval of two years is recommended, although this is not a sufficient criterion to contraindicate uterine testing [25].

For Ruiz [37], 72.5% of dehiscences occur when the delay is less than two years, compared with 27.5% when it is longer.

In order to allow optimal scar consolidation time, patients are advised to space their pregnancies sufficiently. An intergenital space of less than 2 years is not a contraindication to uterine testing. However, a minimum duration of one year remains desirable, given that second-line healing is supposed to take place six months after the operation [37].

1.3.2. Placental insertion

The risk of uterine rupture, as well as the risk of haemorrhage, may be increased when the lower edge of the placenta is located just above the scar. This risk, however, has not been demonstrated in several studies [38].

1.3.3. Uterine overdistension

It is associated with multiple pregnancies, fetal macrosomia or hydramnios.

a. Multiple pregnancy

Most authors consider multiple pregnancy to be a contraindication to uterine testing in previously caesarean patients.

Phelan [39] and his team had authorized uterine testing in a proportion of their patients (45%) with twin pregnancies associated with a scarred uterus, and 72% of these patients delivered normally without any additional maternal-fetal morbidity. It would appear, however, that this approach should be reserved for twin pregnancies in which the first twin is in cephalic apex presentation, in accordance with A.C.O.G. recommendations [16]. Aboulfalah [2] nevertheless performed 62% of maneuvers on the first twin (vacuum, forceps, version by internal maneuver, small assisted extraction and large breech extraction) in a short series of 35 patients. Fetal prognosis was guarded, due to prematurity or hypotrophy, but mortality and perinatal morbidity remained higher in newborns after prophylactic caesarean section, at 8.3% and 12%, than in the group of newborns after uterine challenge, at 6% and 16.6% respectively. Aboulfalah et al [2] found no significant difference in maternal prognosis between the twin and singleton groups.

b. Fetal macrosomia

Excess fetal volume or macrosomia is defined as a birth weight greater than 4000g. [22]

Aboulfalah et al [2] compiled 335 cases of delivery of macrosomic women with scar uteri, with a total of 46.8% Caesarean sections and 53.2% natural vaginal deliveries. There was no significant difference in maternal-fetal prognosis between the prophylactic caesarean section group (16.3%) and the uterine test group (86.7%), even though the risk of uterine rupture increased in parallel with the birth weight of the newborn. In fact, they observed that the success rate of uterine testing decreased significantly with increasing birth weight, from 79.4% for a birth weight of 4,000 g, to 67.4% between 4,000 and 4,500 g, and 47.3% thereafter.

A.C.O.G. guidelines [16] for suspected fetal macrosomia in previously caesareanized patients recommend iterative caesarean section or, at the very least, great caution in authorizing uterine testing.

c. Hydramnios

In the literature, the association of hydramnios with a scarred uterus is an indication for prophylactic caesarean section [40, 41].

1.3.4. Fetal presentation

Classically, any presentation other than cephalic presentation of the vertex in late pregnancy on a scar uterus should be an indication for prophylactic caesarean section. For most authors, vertex presentation is the only presentation that allows uterine testing [25].

Breech version by external manoeuvre is classically contraindicated in previously caesareanized patients, for fear of causing uterine rupture. Phelan et al [39] have shown that this therapeutic approach is possible, without additional maternal-fetal complications.

Having found no significant difference in maternal-fetal prognosis between the cephalic and breech presentation groups, some authors, supported by the A.C.O.G. [16], no longer recommend uterine testing.

1.3.5. Obstetrical ultrasound

It is important to know the strength of the uterine scar, both for the patient's future and for subsequent pregnancies. For this reason, certain paraclinical examinations (such as amniography, which was first proposed in 1972 for the study, during pregnancy, of the scar from a previous caesarean section) can assess the strength of the scar [43]. A defective scar will result in an image of evagination or invagination of the uterine cavity at the level of this scar.

This method was rapidly superseded by ultrasound, which enables the exact thickness of the scar to be measured [30], without risk, during pregnancy:

a. Placental localization.

Low insertion of the placenta on the anterior surface of the uterus, opposite the old scar, is a pejorative element because, by laminating the lower segment, it increases the risk of uterine rupture and placenta accreta, increta or even percreta.

Bromley [44] points out that a placenta previa capable of interposing itself between the bladder and the amniotic cavity may mask a uterine dehiscence. Ultrasound may, therefore, be able to distinguish between the possibility of a hypoechoic inferior segment, very thinned in nature, and a defect of the same tonality.

b. Lower segment study.

As hysterography in the gynaecological period is inconclusive, some authors have proposed obstetrical ultrasound as a means of investigation to identify a predictive factor for uterine rupture.

The main aim seems to be to study the lower segment and identify any dehiscence.

There are 4 ultrasound degrees:

- Grade 1: the scar is not visible.
- Step 2: Localized slimming.
- Grade 3: Scarring bead.
- Grade 4: total scar dehiscence.

Borrowing from this line of research, Michaels [45], in 1988, carried out a case-control study of 70 patients to detect abnormalities of the lower segment of scar uteri on ultrasound. Using a 3.5 MHz probe, he measured the length and thickness of the lower segment, as well as the length of the cervix. In the case of Caesarean section, he compared the ultrasound findings with those of the macroscopic status of the lower segment intraoperatively. He found that there was no significant difference between cases and controls for the parameters of cervical length and lower segment length. Statistically, however, the mean thickness of the lower segment, the distance measured between the chorioamniotic membrane and the muscularis mucosae of the bladder, was significantly different ($p < 0.01$) in patients with lower segment anomalies compared with the control group.

Chapter 2

II. Delivery on scar uterus

The choice of delivery route is guided by the various factors discussed above.

2.1. . High-pressure delivery

In addition to the classic classification, the indications for Caesarean section on scar uterus are grouped into two types:

- Prophylactic caesarean section
- Emergency caesarean section indicated after failure of uterine test

2.2. . Uterine or scar test

2.2.1. . Definition

The uterine test is defined by Lansac [41] as the conduct of vaginal delivery in a scarred uterus. It is therefore a dynamic test, not a "trial of strength".

2.2.2. . Terms and conditions

A number of factors contribute to the choice of vaginal delivery in the case of delivery on a scar uterus. These include

- Segmental anterior Caesarean section,
- The post-operative course is necessarily straightforward,
- The absence of any uterine malformation,
- The absence of maternal pathology against - indicating the vaginal route,
- The absence of overdistension in monofetal pregnancies significant uterine size (uterine height > 38 cm) ruling out any cause other than macrosomia and hydramnios,
- Cephalic presentations of the vertex with a favorable feto-pelvic confrontation,
- A placenta that is not inserted on the scar and the absence of overactive dystocia,

- A hospital of at least secondary level with the conditions and neonatal care,
- The presence of a multidisciplinary medical team including a gynecologist, an anesthesiologist and a pediatric neo-natologist,
- The patient's informed consent to risks incurred during the event.

2.2.3. . Patient care in the delivery room

In the delivery room, the following conditions must be met:

- Establish a complete medical file,
- Perform a full paraclinical workup,
- Pre-anaesthetic visit,
- An available and alert operating room,
- Monitor the fetus continuously by recording the fetal heart rate,
- Monitor uterine contractility with external and then internal tocometry,
- Insert a venous safety line.

During the first two phases of labor, cervical dilation must be regular and harmonious. Any stagnation in dilation calls for an analysis of the situation, based on internal tocometry, in order to distinguish between :

- Possible uterine rupture,
- Dynamic dystocia of the hypokinesia type, to be corrected by oxytocin infusion,
- Cervical dystocia characterized by stagnation of dilation and correct uterine activity: this is the indication for cervical relaxation with antispasmodics or powerful analgesia. If this is not the case, a Caesarean section is required.

The expulsive phase is the most dangerous for the scar, due to the mechanical constraints exerted on it, and instrumental extraction should only be used to shorten it if it lasts more than 20 to 30 minutes. Uterine expression and abdominal press are classically contraindicated.

Delivery is directed in natural deliveries and artificial deliveries in the case of instrumental extraction.

Originally a routine procedure, uterine revision looks for uterine breaches after vaginal delivery. However, it remains an invasive procedure, combining the risk of infection with the risk of anesthesia. According to A.C.O.G. recommendations [16], it should only be performed in the presence of warning signs.

Chapter 3

III. Uterine rupture

This complication should be distinguished from uterine dehiscence, which is often asymptomatic. It is only encountered incidentally, in 0.5 to 2% of elective caesarean sections [47], during uterine testing, and does not expose the mother to any particular maternal-fetal morbidity.

The frequency of uterine rupture during uterine testing is low, barely exceeding 1% [48, 49, 50]. There are usually two categories of uterine rupture:

- Complete ruptures correspond to a tear of the entire thickness of the uterine wall (myometrium and peritoneum), with tearing of the membranes. The consequences for the fetus, and sometimes the mother, can be serious.
- Incomplete rupture or dehiscence, where only the myometrium is torn, leaving the peritoneum and membranes intact. These ruptures, which most often have no maternal-fetal consequences, may be asymptomatic and go unnoticed in the absence of uterine revision.

The risk of uterine rupture appears to be closely related to the type of anterior scar [50, 51].

The use of oxytocin in the active management of labor does not appear to increase the risk of uterine rupture [52, 53].

Epidural analgesia does not increase maternal-fetal risk if monitoring conditions are rigorous and do not mask the possible occurrence of suprapubic pain of uterine rupture [54].

For most authors, cervical ripening with prostaglandin remains formally contraindicated, and this negative opinion is based on a fear of uterine rupture due to uterine hypertonia or hyperkinesia [54].

Fetal complications are dominated by fetal heart rhythm abnormalities in the form of bradycardia or severe variable deceleration, which in most cases represent the first signs of scar dehiscence.

Chapter 4

IV. Conceptual framework

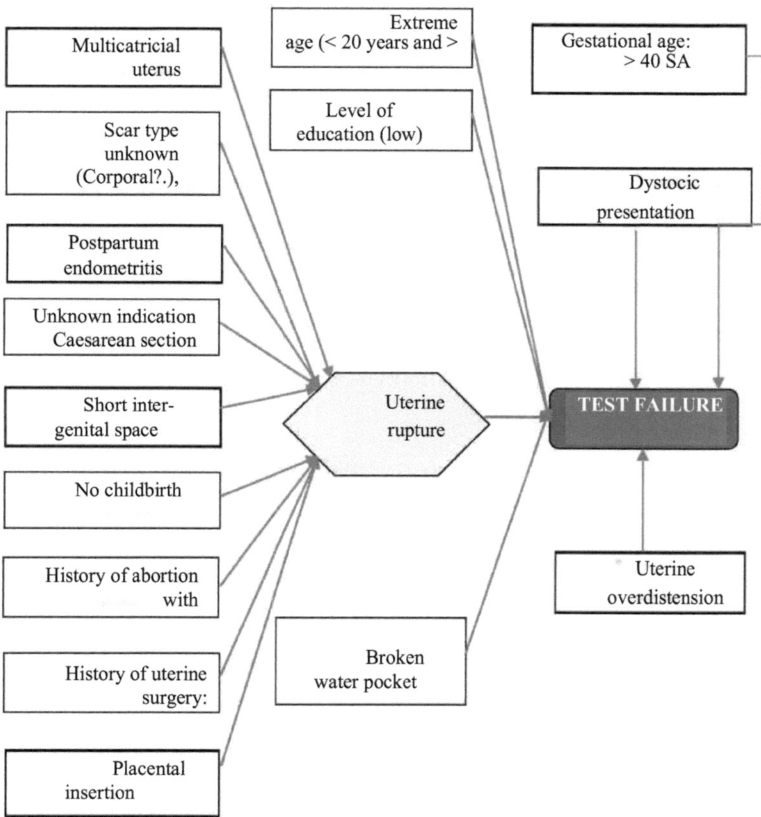

Figure 1: Our conceptual model explaining the occurrence of uterine test failure

PART TWO: PERSONAL OBSERVATIONS
Chapter 1
PATIENTS, MATERIALS AND METHODS

1.1. Operational definitions

1. Patient: a pregnant woman with a scarred uterus, whether in labor or not.
2. Uterine test, also known as the "scar labor test" or "scar test": this is the conduct of a vaginal delivery in a patient with a scar uterus [15].
3. Failed uterine challenge: is any parturition on a scarred uterus that has resulted in maternal-per neonatal morbi - mortality and/or failure to terminate vaginal delivery [15].
4. State of the newborn at birth: is the clinical state of the newborn assessed by measuring the APGAR score at five minutes.
5. Delivery site or Maternity ward: this is the specialized site reserved for deliveries within the 4 hospitals selected for the study.
6. Intergenital interval: the time, in months, between the last Caesarean delivery and the onset of the next pregnancy.

1.2. Type and period of study

Our work is a prospective, multicenter, cross-sectional and analytic study of patients with a scarred uterus who gave birth from January 01, 2013 to December 31, 2013 in the maternity wards of 4 secondary-level referral hospitals in the DRC.

1.3. Geographical and operational characteristics of selected sites

To carry out this study, four maternity units in the DRC's major hospitals were selected on the basis of the following criteria: geographical location, good accessibility, capacity (bed occupancy rate), the presence of at least one obstetrician-gynecologist, an average number of deliveries of at least 80 per month, and the ability to carry out both clinical and paraclinical (laboratory and imaging) diagnoses (Table II).

Table I: Study sites and their operational capacities

N°	Maternity wards	City	No. of beds	No. of Specialists	Average no. of accesses per month
1	HASC	Kinshasa	52	7	86
2	HGRB	Mbuji - Mayi	48	2	133
3	CUL	Lubumbashi	37	8	93
4	SENDWE	Lubumbashi	87	3	175

These hospitals also receive referrals and medical evacuations from other DRC provinces. For the analysis of results, each hospital forms a study group.

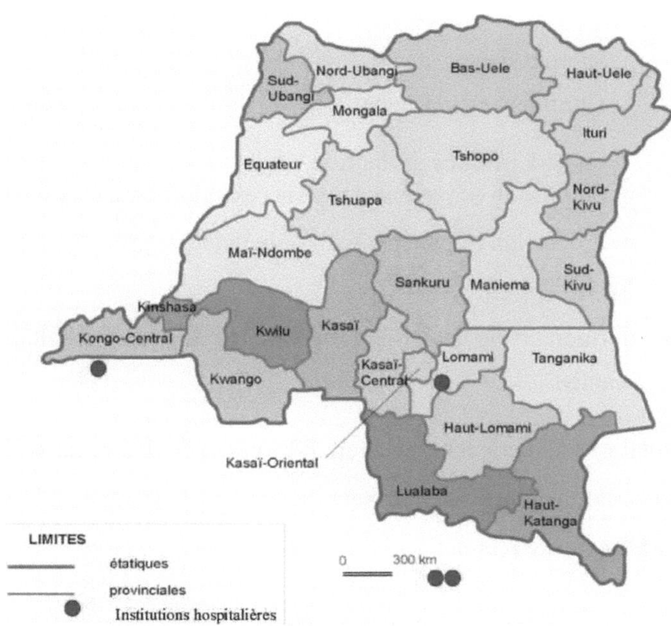

Figure 2: Geographical map of the DRC

1.4. Sampling

1.4.1. Statistical unit

The statistical unit is any patient with a history of caesarean section who attended one of the four maternity units selected.

1.4.2. Sample size and sampling technique

We used exhaustive sampling and consecutive recruitment in hospitals (maternity wards). The minimum sample size was calculated as 290 using the formula below:

$$n \geq \frac{Z_{\alpha}^{2} pq}{d^{2}} \quad n \Rightarrow \frac{(1{,}96)2 \times 0{,}61 \times 0{,}39}{(0.05)2} = 290$$

Where:

- n: Sample size
- Z: Confidence coefficient
- α Risk of error of the first kind
- p: Proportion of patients with successful uterine test: 0.61 [55].
- q: Proportion of patients with failed uterine test (q=100% - p)
- d: Imprecision deviation reflecting the degree of absolute precision wanted.

Of a total of 462 patients registered, 80 were excluded because they did not meet the study criteria or their records were incomplete. In the end, only 382 patients and their newborns were retained.

1.5. Inclusion criteria

The study population comprised patients with a history of caesarean section who met the inclusion criteria below:

- Gestational age > 34 SA
- Mono-fetal pregnancy

- Pregnancy with live fetus
- Previous caesarean section < 2
- No absolute contraindication to vaginal delivery
- Patient with ultrasound performed before 14 SA

1.6. Studied variables

Two variables are dependent in this study: perinatal morbidity and maternal morbidity/mortality. The independent variables were the various patient characteristics. Below are the operational definitions of the different variables:

1.6.1. Socio-demographic characteristics :

- ***Patient age at admission: This is*** a continuous quantitative variable, defined as the completed age at the time of admission to the maternity unit. For our analysis, we defined age ranges as follows: <19 years, 20 - 35 years and >35 years [56].
- ***Level of education:*** This is the level of education attained and reported by the patient at the time of admission. It is a qualitative variable that was subsequently subdivided into 2 modalities: low level (no education, primary) and satisfactory level (secondary, higher and other).
- ***Marital status: This is*** a qualitative variable that determines the patient's marital status. Marital status has been

  Next, divided into 2 categories: living in a union (married, common-law) and living alone (single, divorced, widowed).
- ***The birth attendant's qualifications***: This is a qualitative variable that has been divided into four categories according to the level of academic or schooling achieved:
  - **Specialist**: gynecologist - obstetrician
  - **General practitioner**: doctor of medicine

> **Trainee doctor**: final-year medical student (internship)
> **Nurse/midwife**: nursing staff assigned to the maternity unit, whatever their level.

1.6.2. Clinical characteristics of the patient:

- *Parity:* This is the number of pregnancies reaching at least 22 weeks' amenorrhea (SA) at delivery [56]. In the present study, parity was sorted into two categories before being introduced into the various estimated models: Pauciparity or low parity (2 - 3) and multiparity (> 4).
- *Gestational age:* This was calculated from the specified date of the last menstrual period and/or data from an early ultrasound scan performed before the fourteenth week of amenorrhea. For this quantitative variable, we considered two gestational age groups: 34 S.A - 40 S.A and > 40 S.A.
- *The number of previous caesarean sections:* We have distinguished two classes:

> A uni-scarred uterus with a history of a single caesarean section.
> The bi-cicatricial uterus with the antecedent of two caesarean sections.

- *Indications for previous caesarean section:* These are the non-permanent reasons for deciding on caesarean delivery, and have been grouped into two:

> indications for emergency caesarean section: intrapartum caesarean section indicated after failure of uterine test;
> indications for elective caesarean section: antepartum

caesarean section indicated before any uterine test.

- ***Mode of delivery after last caesarean section: This*** is a qualitative variable, with vaginal delivery and vaginal delivery being the two most common.
- ***Intergenerational interval: This is*** a quantitative variable that has been grouped into two categories: <24 months and >24 months.
- ***Fetal presentation: This is*** a qualitative variable specified by vaginal touch. Only presentations compatible with vaginal delivery are taken into account: cephalic (occipital, bregmatic and facial) and breech.
- ***Degree of cervical dilatation***: This is the degree of opening of the internal orifice of the cervix, assessed by vaginal touch when the patient is admitted.
- ***Labor time (in hours)***: This is the number of labor hours of a delivery counted from the active phase of labor (i.e. from 4 cm dilation to 10 cm). It averages 6 to 10 hours. Prolonged labor [12] is defined as labor lasting more than 10 hours.
- ***Perinatal and maternal development:*** This leads to the following three states*:*
  - > Morbidity (maternal and perinatal) ;
  - > Morbidity-free survival (maternal and perinatal);
  - > Death (maternal or perinatal): before discharge from hospital.

1.7. Collecting data

Patients were seen in the obstetrics departments of the four above-mentioned hospital institutions (prenatal consultations, emergency unit, high-risk obstetrics unit and birthing room).

The data collection form (Appendix 1) was filled in by eight interviewers recruited from the obstetrics staff of the study hospitals. These staff had been trained for 4 days on our research topic and on the data collection procedure.

The material support for the information collected consisted of :

- delivery registers,
- operating report registers,
- partograms,
- neonatal charts, - post-partum hospitalization charts.

1.8. Data processing and analysis

Data were entered on computer using Epi Info 3.5.3, and SPSS 21 software was used for analysis.

The results were presented in the form of tables and graphs. Error bars were used to visualize the mean and confidence interval of the various quantitative variables with an approximately normal distribution. The mean with its standard deviation was calculated for normally distributed quantitative variables, or the median with its interquartile range for non-normally distributed variables. The proportion for qualitative variables with a 95% confidence interval has been calculated.

Student's t-test was used to compare the means of the four groups in pairs. Single-factor ANOVA was used to compare the means of at least three groups, and post hoc tests were used to compare multiple means. The Chi-square test with Yates correction and, if necessary, Fisher's exact test were used to compare small frequencies.

Bi-variate analyses were used to identify factors associated with poor maternal-fetal prognosis. The logistic regression model was used to identify the determinants of perinatal and maternal morbidity. In both cases, only variables with a significance level less than or equal to 0.10 were considered. Adjusted odds ratios and their 95% confidence intervals were used to assess the strength of the various associations sought. The logistic regression model was further constructed to identify the determinants of uterine test failure. Only variables with a p-value < 0.05

and less likely to be subjective were included in the model analysis.

1.9. Ethical considerations.

Before collecting the data, we had to obtain the approval of the ethics committee of the University of Lubumbashi (Appendix 2), to whom we explained the objectives and methodology of the study.

The data were collected anonymously, and the information presented in this work does not contain any element that could allow the identification of the subjects or their children, who gave their free, informed and verbal consent after explanation of the objectives of the study. The data collection forms were given to the principal investigator, who kept them until the end of data collection. After data entry and cleaning of the database, all patient files were kept securely in the various maternity units.

While there was no direct benefit for the participants in this study, it will enable future perspectives to be developed, so as to improve the management of patients with scar uteri.

Chapter 2

RESULTS

11.1. FREQUENCY OF DELIVERIES ON SCARRED UTERI, TERMINATION ROUTES AND MORBIDITY - MATERNAL AND PERINATAL MORTALITY

11.1.1. Frequency of deliveries on scar uteri

During the study period, the 4 maternity units recorded 5854 deliveries, 382 of which were on scar uteri, giving an overall rate of 6.53%. The highest frequency was reported at Hôpital de l'Amitié Sino - Congolaise in Kinshasa (10.81%), and the lowest at Hôpital SENDWE (3.71%), with a statistically significant difference (p=0.00), (table III).

Table II: Rates of delivery on scarred uteri, by study site

Sites	No. deliveries total *N*	No. of scarred uteruses *n*	*%*	*p*
HASC	1036	112	10,81	-
CUL	1118	64	5,72	0,00001
SENDWE	2100	78	3,71	0,00000
HGRB	1600	128	8,00	0,01
TOTAL	***5854***	***382***	***6,53***	

I.2 Socio-demographic, clinical and obstetrical characteristics

The average age of the patients was 31. 28±7 .38 years, with more under 20 years of age at the Hôpital Général de Référence de BIMPEBA in Mbuji - Mayi (p=0.003). On the other hand, there were significantly more patients living alone at Hôpital de l'Amitié Sino-Congolaise and Cliniques Universitaires de Lubumbashi than at Hôpital SENDWE de Lubumbashi and Hôpital Général de Référence de BIMPEBA (p=0.007). The proportion of educated patients was statistically higher at SENDWE and Hôpital Général de Référence de BIMPEBA than at Cliniques Universitaires de Lubumbashi and Hôpital de l'Amitié Sino-Congolaise (p=0.02). Mean parity ranged from 3.6 ±1 .5 in Kinshasa to 4.4 ± 2.1 in Lubumbashi.

(SENDWE) with an overall mean of 4.0 ± 2.0, and more primiparous at the BIMPEMBA General Referral Hospital (p=0.014). Just over 20% of uterine scars were under 13 months of age at SENDWE and BIMPEMBA, compared with around 15% at the Cliniques Universitaires de Lubumbashi and Hôpital de l'Amitié Sino-Congolaise, with no statistically significant difference. The same applies to the condition of fetal membranes on admission, but the difference was only significant between the Cliniques Universitaires de Lubumbashi and the Hôpital Général de Référence de BIMPEMBA (p=0.004). (Tables IV and V).

Table III: Socio-demographic characteristics of patients by delivery site

Features	HASC n=112	CUL n=64	P	SENDWE n=78	p	HGRB n=128	P
Maternal age (years)							
< 20 n = 25 (6,54)	3 (2,7)	1 (1,6)		4 (5,1)		17(13,3)	
20-35 n= 220 (57,8)	67(59.8)	36 (56.3)		49 (620.8)		68(53.1)	
> 35 n= 137 (35.86)	42(37.5)	27 (42.2)	1.000	25 (32.1)	0.448	43 (336)	0.003
Education level							
Low n=182 (47.6)	63(56.2)	36 (56.2)		29 (37.2)		54(42.2)	
Satisfactory n= 200 (52,5)	49(43.8)	28 (43.8)	1.000	49 (62.8)	0.009	74(57.8)	0.02
Marital status							
In union n= 277 (72,5)	69(61.61)	48(75.0)		61 (78.21)		99(77.37)	
Living alone n= 105 (27.5)	43(38.39)	16 (25.0)	0.070	17 (21.79)	0.015	29(22.66)	0.007

Table IV: Clinical and obstetric characteristics of patients by delivery site

Table IV shows the clinical and obstetric characteristics of patients by delivery site.

Features	**HASC** n=112	**CUL** n=64	p	**SENDWE** n=78	p	**HGRB** n=128	p
Parity							
Primipare n=28 (7,33)	5 (4.5)	3 (4.7)		2 (2.6)		18 (14.1)	
Paucipare n= 147 (38,48)	49(43.7)	27(42.2)		30 (38.5)		41 (32.0)	
Multipare n= 156 (40,84)	52(46.04)	21(32.8)		30 (38.5)		53 (41.4)	
Large multiparous n= 51 (13,35)	6 (5.4)	13 (20.3)	1.000	16 (20.5)	0.702	16 (12.5)	0.014
Last C-section							
< 13 months n=69 (18,06)	16(14,29)	11(17,18)		16(20,51)		26 (20,31)	
13-24 months n=253 (66,23)	86(76,79)	38(59,38)		49(62,82)		80 (62,50)	
>24 months n=60(15,71)	10 (8,93)	15(23,44)	0.410	13(16,67)	0.062	22 (17,19)	0.298
Low route after last caesarean section							
No n=209 (54,71)	74 (66.1)	38 (59.4)		38 (48.7)		59 (46.1)	
Yes n=173 (45,29)	38 (33.9)	26 (40.6)	0.374	40 (51.3)	0.016	69 (53.9)	0.001
Gestational age (SA)		-					
34- 40 n=65 (17,02)	24(20,87)	18(26,87)		11 (14,10)		12 (4,92)	
> 40 n=323 (84,55)	88(79,13)	46(73,13)	0,317	67(85,90)	0,201	116(95,08)	0.009
Membrane condition							
Intact n=229 (59,95)	70 (62,5)	36(56,25)		40(51,28)		83 (64,84)	
Broken n=153 (40,05)	42 (37,5)	28 (43,75)	0,416	38 (48,72)	0,12	45 (35,16)	0,71

1.3. Birth attendant qualifications

Table V: Birth attendant qualifications by delivery site

Birth attendant qualifications	HASC n=112 (10,81%)	SENDWE n=78 (3,71%)	CUL n=64 5,72%	HGRB n=128 (8,00%)	Set	p
Specialists	6 (5,4)	5 (6,4)	4 (6,3)	4 (3,1)	19 (5,0)	0,001
General practitioners	25 (22,3)	25 (32,1)	17 26,6)	40(31,3)	107 (28,0)	
Trainee doctors	37 (33,0)	18 (23,1)	15 23,4)	10 (7,8)	80(20,9)	
Nurses/accoucheuses	44 (39,3)	30 (38,4)	28(43,7)	74(57,8)	176(46,1)	

Table VI shows that 6% of deliveries in Lubumbashi (SENDWE and CUL) were directed by specialists, compared with the other two sites (p=0.001), while at BIPEMBA General Referral Hospital the majority of deliveries were directed by nurses and/or birth attendants.

1.4. Methods of delivery on scar uteri.

1.4.1. Delivery route

Table VII shows the outcome of scar uterus deliveries by delivery site.

Table VI: AUC outcome by delivery site

Modes exit	HASC n=112 (10,81%)	CUL n=64 (5,72%)	p	SENDWE n=78 (3,71%)	p	HGRB n=128 (8,00%)	P
TAVB n=365 95,55) (							
Success n = 183(50,14)	45(43,69)	28(44,44)		32(43,84)		78(61,9)	0,013
Failure n=182 (49,86)	58(56,31)	35(55,56)	0,924	41(56,16)	0,984	48(38,0)	0.006
Cesarean section elective n=17(4,45)	9 (8, 04)	1 (1,56)	0,095	5(6,41)	0,673	2(1,56)	0.016

Nearly half the patients delivered vaginally, with only the BIPEMBA General Referral Hospital performing fewer caesarean sections than other sites (p=0.001), (table VII).

1.4.2. Working hours

The duration of labor ranged from 3 to 72 hours for patients who delivered vaginally. The median duration of labor was 8 hours, with an interquartile range of 3 hours. For patients who had a vaginal delivery, the duration of uterine testing prior to the decision to caesarean section ranged from 3 to 48 hours. This duration was shorter at Hôpital de l'Amitié Sino-Congolaise than at other delivery sites (Table VIII).

Table VII: Median duration of labor by delivery site

Working hours	**HASC**	**CUL**	**SENDWE**	**HGRB**
Median duration (Q1, Q3)	7 (6, 8)	10 (8,12)	10 (8,12)	10 (8,12)
Minimum duration	3	3	3	3
Maximum duration	10	72	48	48

4.4.3. Indications of last caesarean delivery

Table VIII: Indications of last cesarean delivery and type of cesarean delivery

Types of Caesarean section	**Indications**	**n**	**%**
Emergency Caesarean section	Pre-break ring	34	17,09
	Eclampsia	2	1,01
	Cervical dystocia	8	4,02
	Dynamic dystocia resistant to treatment	8	4,02
	DPPNI	4	2,01
	Prolonged work	1	0,50
	Circular cord	3	1,51
	Macrosomia	1	0,50
	Failure to commit	14	7,04
	Vice de présentation	7	3,52
	SFA	41	20,60
	Placenta previa	18	9,05
	Procidence of the cord	3	1,51
	Uterine rupture	38	19,10
	Subtotal	**182**	**91,46**
Elective Caesarean	Boundary basin	9	4,52

section			
	Pre-eclampsia	1	0,50
	Macrosomia	1	0,50
	Cross-functional presentation	2	1,01
	Placenta previa	4	2,01
	Subtotal	**17**	**8,54**
	Total	**199**	**100**

Table IX shows a high proportion of emergency caesarean sections, i.e. 91.5%, compared with 8.5% for elective caesarean sections. The highest frequencies of indications are represented respectively by acute fetal distress with 41 cases (20.60%), uterine rupture with 38 cases (19.10%), pre-rupture ring with 34 cases (17.09%) and placenta previa with 18 cases (9.05%).

1.5. Anthropometric parameters of newborns

Table X reports the anthropometric parameters of newborns - by delivery site.

Table IX: Anthropometric parameters of newborns - by delivery site

Features	HASC	CUL	SENDWE	HGRB
Weight	3161±619	3461±554	3302±467	3327±466
Size	51.1±1.4	51.2±1.6	50.9±1.3	50.6±2.6
Cranial perimeter	34.5±2.3	34.6±3.7	34.3±1.5	34.5±1.5

Mean newborn birth weight was 3313 ± 528 g overall (p=0.004), mean height 51 ± 2 cm for all sites (p=0.096), and mean head circumference 34 ± 2 cm for all four delivery sites (p=0.932).

1.6. Evolution parameters

1.6.1. Maternal morbidity and mortality

Table XI reports maternal morbidity and mortality in deliveries with scar uterus, by delivery site.

Table X: Morbi - AUC maternal mortality by delivery site

Features	HASC	CUL	SEND WE	HGRB

	n=112 (10,81%)	n=64 (5,72%)	p	n=78 (3,71%)	p	n=128 (8,00%)	p
Maternal morbidity							
Absent n= 303 (79.32)	93 (83.04)	48(75.00)		71(91.3)		91 (71.09)	
Present n= 79 (20.68)	19 (16.96)	16(25.00)	0.198	7(8.97)	0.114	37 (28.91)	0.029
Hemorrhage n=33 (8.64)	8 (7.14)	5 (7.31)	0.870	2(2.56)	0.202	18(14.06)	0.085
Uterine rupture n= 6 (1.57)	1 (0.89)	1 (1.56)	1.000	2 (2.56)	0.568	2 (1.56)	1.000
Infection n= 27 (7.07)	7 (6.25)	5 (7.81)	0.692	2 (2.56)	0.312	13 (10.16)	0.274
Other n= 13 (3.40)	3 (2.68)	5 (7.81)		1 (1.28)		4 (3.12)	
Maternal mortality							
Deaths n=5 (1,31)	1 (0.89)	1 (1.56)		2 (2.56)		1 (0.78)	
Survival n= 377 (98.69)	111(99.11)	63(98.44)	1.000	76(97.44)	0.569	127(99.22)	1.000

With a rate of 20.68%, morbidity was dominated by haemorrhage and infection (p=0.73). Complication rates ranged from 8.97% in SENDWE to 28.91% in BIPEMBA, where the risk was doubled compared with other sites (OR: 2.05 [1.23 - 3.40]). Uterine rupture was diagnosed in 6 deliveries (1.57%), with no statistically significant difference between sites (p=1.000). Overall, 5 cases of maternal mortality were recorded, with no statistical difference between sites or delivery route.

1.6.2. Neonatal morbidity and mortality

Table XII reports the perinatal morbidity and mortality of scar uterus deliveries by delivery site.

Table XI: Morbi - perinatal mortality in AUCs

Features	HASC n=112	CUL n=64	p	SEND WE	HGRB	P

	(10,81%)	(5,72%)		n=78 (3,71%)	p	n=128 (8,00%)	
Score of APGAR							
APGAR < 7 147(37.2)	66 (58.9)	33 (51)		25 (32.1)		23 (18)	
APGAR > 7 235(62.8)	46 (42.2)	31(49.2)	0.373	53 (68.8)	0.0003	105(84.0)	0.0000
Mortality Neonatal							
Deaths n=31 (8,2)	4 (3.757)	5 (7.80)		9 (11.54)		13 (10.46)	
Survival n=351(91,8)	108(96.43)	59(92.19)	0.220	69(88.46)	0.037	115(89.84)	0.044

An APGAR score < 7 concerned 147 newborns, with a predominance at Hôpital de l'Amitié Sino-Congolaise and Cliniques Universitaires de Lubumbashi compared with the other two sites (p=0.000). On the other hand, neonatal mortality was low in the first two sites combined (p=0.047).

11. 2. DETERMINANTS OF FETO-MATERNAL OUTCOME AND UTERINE TEST

BIVARIATE ANALYSES

11.1.1. Socio-demographic factors and uterine testing

Table XII: Patient socio-demographic factors associated with uterine test failure

Characteristics	Total	Uterine test *Failure*	*Success*	OR gross (IC95%)	P
Age (years)					
< 20	23 (100)	16 (69,6)	7 (30,4)	2,64 (1,04 - 6,67)	0,041
20 - 35	211 (100)	98 (46,4)	113(53,6)	1	
> 35	131 (100)	78 (59,5)	53 (40,5)	1,70 (1,10 - 2,64)	0,019
Website					
CUL	63 (100)	37 (58,7)	26 (41,3)	1,90(1,03 - 3,50)	0,04
HASC	103 (100)	60 (58,3)	43 (41,7)	1,86(1,10 - 3,15)	0,02
SENDWE	73 (100)	41 (56,2)	32 (43,8)	1,71(0,96 - 3,06)	0,07
HGRB	126 (100)	54 (42,9)	72 (57,1)	1	
Education level					

Low	172 (100)	98 (57,0)	74 (43,0)	1,40 (0,92 -2,11)	0,114
Good	193 (100)	94 (48,7)	99 (51,3)	1	
Marital status					
In union	265(100)	153(57,7)	112(42,3)	2,14(1,34 - 3,42)	0,001
Living alone	100(100)	39(39,0)	61(61,0)	1	

Of the various socio-demographic factors, only patient age, marital status and delivery site were significantly associated with uterine test outcome. In fact, patients in union were 2 times more likely to experience a failed uterine test (OR: 2.14 95% CI: 1.34 - 3.42) than those living alone. Compared with patients aged between 20 and 35, those under 20 and over 35 were more likely to experience uterine test failure. As for the delivery site, the BIMPEMBA General Reference Hospital, with 43%, recorded fewer uterine test failures than the other sites, where proportions in excess of 55% were recorded (Table XIII).

11.1.2. Obstetrical factors and uterine testing

Of all the patients' obstetrical factors, only parity and previous abortion were significantly associated with uterine test outcome. Indeed, patients with a parity greater than 4 were twice as likely to have a failed uterine test (OR: 1.66 95% CI: 1.10 - 2.51) than those with a parity less than 4. Patients with a history of abortion were 5 times more likely to experience uterine test failure (OR: 5.26 95% CI: 2.38 - 11.61) than those with no history of abortion (Table XIV).

Table XIII: Patient obstetrical factors associated with uterine test failure

Features	**Total**	**Uterine test** *Failure*	*Success*	**Crude OR (IC95%)**	**p**
Parity					
-< 4	170(100)	78 (45,9)	92 (54,1)	1	
-> 4	195 (100)	114 (58,5)	81 (41,5)	1,66 (1,10 -2,51)	0,017
Previous abortion					
- No	318 (100)	153 (48,1)	165 (51,9)	1	
-Yes	47 (100)	39 (83,0)	8 (17,0)	5,26 (2,38 -11,61)	< 0,001
Intergenerational space (months)					
-> 24	45 (100)	20 (44,4)	25 (55,6)	1	
-< 24	320 (100)	172 (53,8)	148 (46,2)	1,45 (0,78 - 2,72)	0,244

11.1.3. Clinical factors and uterine testing

In terms of patient clinical factors, only the condition of the water bag and fetal presentation were significantly associated with uterine test outcome. Patients admitted with a ruptured water bag were 5 times more likely to have a failed uterine test (OR: 4.76 95% CI: 2.86 - 7.92) than those admitted with an intact water bag. Non-cephalic presentations of the vertex were 5 times more associated with uterine test failure (OR: 4.80 95% CI: 2.88-8.00) (Table XV).

Table XIV: Patient clinical factors associated with uterine test failure

Features	Total	Uterine test		Crude OR (IC95%)	P
		FailureSuc	*cess*		
Water pocket					
- Broken	116(100)	89 (76,7)	27 (23,3)	4,76 (2,86 - 7,92)	< 0,001
- Intact	215 (100)	88 (40,9)	127 (59,1)	1	
Presentation					
- Summit	254 (100)	106 (41,7)	148 (58,3)	1	
- Others	111 (100)	86 (77,5)	25 (22,5)	4,80 (2,88 - 8,00)	< 0,001

11.1.4. Maternal and neonatal morbidity and risk factors *Table XV: Socio-demographic characteristics of patients and maternal morbidity.*

Features	Maternal morbidity		Crude OR (IC95%)
	Yes	*No*	
Age (years)			
-< 20	4 (11,4)	31 (88,6)	1
-20 - 35	44 (21,6)	160 (78,4)	2,13 (0,71 - 6,36)
-> 35	30 (21,0)	113 (79,0)	2,06 (0,67 - 6,28)
Education level			
-Low	40 (22,0)	142 (78,0)	1,20 (0,73 - 1,98)
-Good	38 (19,0)	162 (81,0)	1
Marital status			
-Living alone	20 (19,0)	85 (81,0)	0,89 (0,50- 1,57)
-In union	58 (20,9)	219 (79,1)	1
Birth attendant qualifications			
- General practitioner	24 (22,4)	83 (77,6)	1,08 (0,34- 4,11)
- Trainee doctor	21 (26,3)	59 (73,8)	1,33 (0,41 - 5,13)
- Nurse/accoucheuse	29 (16,5)	147 (83,5)	0,74 (0,24 - 2,76)
- Specialist	4 (21,1)	15 (78,9)	1
Site*			
-HASC	20 (17,9)	92 (82,1)	2,10 (0,80 - 5,54)

-HGRB	35 (27,3)	93 (72,7)	3,64 (1,44 - 9,18)
-SENDWE	17 (21,8)	61 (78,2)	2,69 (0,99 - 7,31)
-CUL	6 (9,4)	58 (90,6)	1

* : statistically significant characteristics

Table XVI: Clinical and obstetric characteristics of patients and maternal morbidity.

Features	Maternal morbidity Yes	No	Crude OR (IC95%)
Parity			
-> 4	38 (18,4)	169 (81,6)	0,76 (0,46 - 1,25)
-< 4	40 (22,9)	135 (77,1)	1
Intergenerational space* (IGS)			
-> 24 months	13 (35,1)	24 (64,9)	2,82 (1,34 - 5,94)
-< 24 months	47 (16,1)	245 (83,9)	1
Delivery route			
-Cesarean section	47 (23,6)	152 (76,4)	1,52 (0,91 - 2,52)
-Low	31 (16,9)	152 (83,1)	1
Uterine height (cm)			
-> 34	19 (19,8)	77 (80,2)	0,97 (0,54 - 1,74)
-< 34	53 (20,3)	208 (79,7)	1

Tables XVI and XVII show that patients' socio-demographic, clinical and obstetrical characteristics were not associated with maternal morbidity, with the exception of delivery site and intergenital interval. A proportion of maternal morbidity of 35% was recorded among patients with an intergenital interval of less than 24 months, compared with only 16% among those with an interval of more than 24 months (p=0.005). In terms of delivery site, the proportion of morbidity was lowest at the Cliniques Universitaires de Lubumbashi (9%), compared with 18%, 27% and 22% respectively at Hôpital de l'Amitié Sino-Congolaise, Hôpital Général de Référence de BIMPEMBA and SENDWE.

11.2.5. Maternal characteristics and perinatal morbidity

Table XVIII shows the socio-demographic characteristics of patients associated with perinatal morbidity.

Table XVII: Socio-demographic characteristics of patients and perinatal

morbidity

Features	**Perinatal morbidity**		**Crude OR**	
	Yes	***No***	**(IC95%)**	**p**
Age (years)				
-< 20	3 (12,5)	21 (87,5)	1	
-20 - 35	84 (39,3)	130 (60,7)	4,52 (1,31 - 15,64)	0,017
->35	52 (38,2)	84 (61,8)	4,33 (1,23 - 15,25)	0,022
Education level				
-Low	89 (50,0)	89 (50,0)	2,92 (1,89 - 4,51)	< 0,001
-Good	50 (25,5)	146 (74,5)	1	
Marital status				
-Living alone	43 (42,2)	59 (57,3)	1,34 (0,84 - 2,13)	0,222
-In Union	96 (35,3)	176 (64,7)	1	
Site*				
-HGRB	20 (16,0)	105 (84,0)	1	
-HASC	63 (57,8)	46 (42,2)	7,19 (3,90 - 13,24)	< 0,001
-SENDWE	24 (31,2)	53 (68,8)	2,38 (1,21 - 4,69)	0,012
-CUL	32 (50,8)	31 (49,2)	5,42 (2,73 - 10,78)	< 0,001

Table XVIII: Clinical and obstetrical characteristics of patients and perinatal morbidity

Features	Perinatal morbidity		Crude OR (IC95%)	p
	Yes	No		
Parity				
-< 4	59 (34,3)	110 (65,1)	1	
-> 4	80 (39,0)	125 (61,0)	1,19 (0,78 - 1,82)	0,413
Intergenerational space (months)				
-< 24	108 (38,0)	176 (62,0)	1,91(0,87 - 4,20)	0,108
-> 24	9 (24,3)	28 (75,7)	1	
Delivery route				
-Low	44 (24,6)	135 (75,4)	2,92 (1,88 - 4,53)	< 0,001
-Cesarean section	95 (48,7)	100 (51,3)	1	
Uterine height (cm)				
-< 34	100 (39,1)	156 (60,9)	1	
-> 34	66 (69,5)	29 (30,5)	0,68 (0,41 - 1,13)	0,142
Membrane condition				
-Intact	63 (29,0)	154 (71,0)	1	
-Broken	52 (42,6)	70 (57,4)	1,82 (1,14 - 2,89)	0,012
Pregnancy pathology during pregnancy				
-Present	24 (34,3)	46 (65,7)	0,86 (0,50 - 1,48)	0,58
-Absent	115 (37,8)	189 (62,2)	1	

Prematurity				
-No	28 (58,3)	20 (41,7)	1	
-Yes	111 (35,5)	202 (64,5)	2,55 (1,37 - 4,73)	0,003

Tables XVIII and XIX show that only maternal age, the patient's level of education, the route of delivery, the condition of the water sac on admission and the delivery site were statistically associated with perinatal morbidity. Indeed, a higher proportion of perinatal morbidity was recorded among patients aged over 35 (OR: 4.33; CI95%: 1.23 - 15.25; p= 0.022) and even among those aged between 20 and 35 (p=0.017). In addition, 43% of perinatal morbidity was recorded in patients admitted with a ruptured water bag, compared with only 29% in those admitted with an intact water bag (p=0.012). The HASC (58%) and the Cliniques Universitaires de LUBUMBASHI (51%) recorded higher proportions of perinatal mortality, compared with the Hopital Général de Référence de BIMPEMBA (16%) and SENDWE (31%).

II.1.6. Maternal characteristics and perinatal mortality

Table XIX: Socio-demographic characteristics of patients and perinatal mortality

Features	Perinatal mortality		Crude OR	
	Yes	*No*	(IC95%)	P
Age (years)				
-< 20	0 (0)	24 (100)	0,26 (0,01 - 1,76)	0,283
-20 - 35	21 (9,9)	192 (90,1)	1	
-> 35	10 (7,5)	124 (92,5)	0,75 (0,32 - 1,76)	0,603
Education level				
-Low	14 (7,9)	163 (82,1)	0,89 (0,43 - 1,87)	0,767
-Good	17 (8,8)	177 (91,2)	1	
Marital status				
-Living alone	7 (6,8)	96 (83,2)	0,74 (0,31 - 1,78)	0,501
-In union	24 (8,9)	244(81,1)	1	
Birth attendant qualifications				
- General practitioners	10 (9,5)	95 (90,5)	0,89 (0,18 - 9,12)	0,998
- Trainee doctors	13 (16,7)	65 (83,3)	1,69 (0,33 - 16,87)	0,795
- Nurse/accoucheuse	6 (3,5)	163 (96,5)	0,32 (0,05 - 3,44)	0,375
- Specialist physicians	2 (10,5)	17 (89,5)	1	
Site*				
-HASC	4 (3,7)	105 (96,3)	1	

-HGRB	13 (10,4)	112 (89,6)	3,05 (0,96 - 9,64)	0,047
-SENDWE	9 (11,8)	67 (88,2)	3,53 (1,04 - 11,91)	0,032
-CUL	5 (8,2)	56 (91,8)	2,33 (0,48 - 12,24)	0,362

* : statistically significant characteristics

Table XX: Clinical and obstetrical characteristics of patients and perinatal mortality

	Perinatal mortality			**p**
Features	*Yes*	*No*	**Crude OR (IC95%)**	
Parity				
-< 4	9 (5,4)	159 (94,6)	1	
-> 4	22 (10,8)	181 (89,2)	2,14 (0,96 - 4,86)	0,057
Intergenerational space (months)				
-< 24	19 (6,8)	262 (83,2)	0,59 (0,18 - 2,57)	0,543
-> 24	4 (10,8)	33 (89,2)	1	
Delivery route				
-Low	7 (3,9)	169 (96,1)	1	
-Cesarean section	24 (12,3)	171 (87,7)	0,60 (0,18 - 2,57)	0,544
Uterine height (cm)				
-< 34	24 (9,4)	231(90,6)	1	
-> 34	6 (6,4)	88 (93,6)	0,66 (0,26 - 1,66)	0,371
Membrane condition				
-Intact	11 (36,7)	205 (67,0)	1	
-Broken	19 (63,3)	101 (33,0)	3,51 (1,61 - 7,65)	0,002
Pregnancy pathology during pregnancy				
-Present	11 (15,7)	59 (84,3)	2,62 (1,19 - 5,76)	0,014
-Absent	20 (6,6)	281 (93,4)	1	
Prematurity				
-No	28 (9,1)	281(90,9)	0,64 (0,12 - 2,21)	0,692
-Yes	3 (6,0)	47 (94,0)	1	

The only factors statistically associated with perinatal mortality were: parity, status of the water sac on admission, presence of gravid pathology during pregnancy and site of delivery. A higher proportion of perinatal mortality was recorded among patients with a parity of at least 4 (10.8 vs. 5.4; p= 0.057). Furthermore, 63% of perinatal mortality cases were recorded among patients admitted with a ruptured water bag, compared with only 37% of patients admitted with an intact water bag (p=0.002). With regard to pathology during pregnancy, 15.7% of perinatal mortality cases were observed in patients with gravid pathology during pregnancy, compared with only 6.6% in patients without gravid pathology (p= 0.014). The Hôpital Général de Référence de BIPEMBA (10%)

and SENDWE (12%) recorded higher proportions of perinatal mortality, compared with the Cliniques Universitaires de Lubumbashi (8%) and HASC (4%).

11.3. MULTIVARIATE ANALYSIS

11.3.1. Maternal characteristics and perinatal morbidity

Table XXII shows the socio-demographic, clinical and obstetrical characteristics of patients associated with perinatal morbidity.

Table XXI: Maternal characteristics and perinatal morbidity

Features	Crude OR (IC95%)	P	Adjusted OR (IC95%)	P
Age (years)				
-< 20	1		1	
-20 - 35	4,52(1,31 - 15,64)	0,017	20,07(2,01- 200,18)	0,011
-> 35	4,33(1,23 - 15,25)	0,022	19,71(1,93 - 301,69)	0,012
Education level				
-Low	2,92(1,89 - 4,51)	< 0,001	3,74(2,04 - 6,86)	< 0,001
-Good	1		1	
Delivery route				
-Low	1		1	
- Cesarean section	2,92 (1,88 - 4,53)	<0,001	0,48 (0,24 - 0,92)	0,027
Membrane condition				
-Intact	1		1	
-Broken	1,82(1,14 - 2,89)	0,012	1,92(1,00 - 3,69)	0,05
Prematurity				
-No	1		1	
-Yes	2,55(1,37 - 4,73)	0,003	0,52(0,23 - 1,16)	0,109
Website				
-HGRB	1		1	
-HASC	7,19(3,90 - 13,24)	< 0,001	6,95(2,92 - 16,57)	< 0,001
-SENDWE	2,38(1,21 - 4,69)	0,012	2,56(1,01 -6,42)	0,046
-CUL	5,42(2,73 - 10,78)	< 0,001	4,73(1,85 - 12,12)	0,001

After adjustment with logistic regression, delivery site, membrane status, route of delivery, education level and patient age were significantly associated with perinatal morbidity. Compared with BIPEMBA General Reference Hospital (16%), the risk of perinatal morbidity was 2.56 times higher at Sendwe (31.2%),

4.73 times higher at CUL (50.8%) and 6.95 times higher at Hôpital de l'Amitié Sino-Congolaise (57.8%). Ruptured membranes (42.6%) presented 1.92 times more risk than intact membranes (29%). Caesarean section (48.7%) was 2.92 times more risky than vaginal delivery (24.6%). The risk associated with a low level of education (50%) was 3.74 times greater than that associated with a high level of education (25.5%). Compared with patients aged under 20 (12.5%), those aged 20 - 35 (39.3%) and over 35 (38.2%) had a 20.07 and 19.71 times greater risk respectively (table XXII).

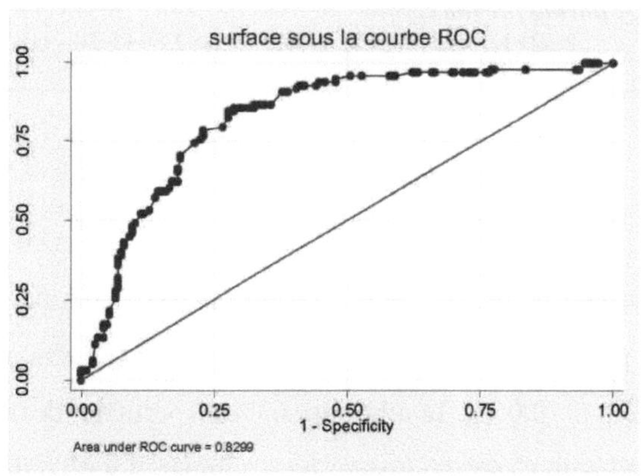

Figure 3: Goodness-of-fit test of the perinatal morbidity model

The area under the ROC curve of the estimated model is 83%, which would mean that the estimated model has good predictive power, with a sensitivity of 59%, a specificity of 85%, a positive predictive value of 68% and a negative predictive value of 80%. This predicted model enabled 80% of newborns to be correctly classified.

II.3.2 Maternal characteristics and perinatal mortality

Table XXIII shows the socio-demographic, clinical and obstetrical characteristics of patients associated with perinatal mortality.

Table XXII: Maternal characteristics and perinatal mortality

Features	Crude OR (IC95%)	P	Adjusted OR (IC95%)	P
Parity				
-< 4	1			
-> 4	2,14 (0,96 - 4,86)	0,057	2,44 (1,02 - 5,87)	0,046
Membrane condition				
-Intact	1		1	
-Broken	3,51(1,61 - 7,65)	0,002	3,82 (1,67 - 8,71)	0,001
Pregnancy pathology during pregnancy				
- Present	2,62 (1,19 - 5,76)	0,014	2,87 (1,20 - 6,85)	0,017
-Absent	1		1	
Website				
-HASC	1		1	
-HGRB	3,05 (0,96 - 9,64)	0,047	3,59 (0,88 - 14,59)	0,074
-SENDWE	3,53 (1,04 - 11,91)	0,032	2,95 (0,64 - 13,53)	0,164
-CUL	2,33 (0,48 - 12,24)	0,362	3,07 (0,82 - 11,51)	0,096

In the bivariate analysis, a higher proportion of perinatal mortality was recorded among patients with a parity of at least 4 (10.8% vs. 5.4% among multiparous women; p= 0.057). In addition, 63% of perinatal deaths were recorded in patients admitted with a ruptured water bag, compared with only 37% in patients admitted with an intact water bag (p=0.002). As for gravidic pathologies, 15.7% of perinatal mortality cases were observed in patients who had experienced a gravidic pathology during pregnancy, compared with only 6.6% in patients with no notion of gravidic pathology (p= 0.014). In Mbuji - Mayi, the Hôpital Général de Référence de BIMPEBA (10%) and the Hôpital SENDWE de Lubumbashi (12%) recorded higher proportions of perinatal mortality than the Cliniques Universitaires de Lubumbashi (8%) and the Hôpital de l'Amitié Sino - Congolais de Kinshasa (4%).

In the multivariate analysis and after adjustment with logistic regression, we observed :

1) multiparous women were 2.44 times more likely to see their child die during the perinatal period than those with a parity of less than 4;

2) patients with premature rupture of membranes were 4 times more likely to see their child die during the perinatal period;
3) patients with pregnancy-related pathology were 3 times more likely to see their child die during the perinatal period;

As for the delivery site, patients attended at the Hôpital Général de Référence de BIPEMBA were 4 times more likely, and those attended at the Cliniques Universitaires de Lubumbashi were 3 times more likely, to see their child die during the perinatal period than those who gave birth at Hôpital de l'Amitié Sino-Congolaise.

4) but the difference observed was not statistically significant at the a=0.05 threshold. All the differences observed, except for the geographical locations of the hospitals (sites), were statistically significant (table XXIII).

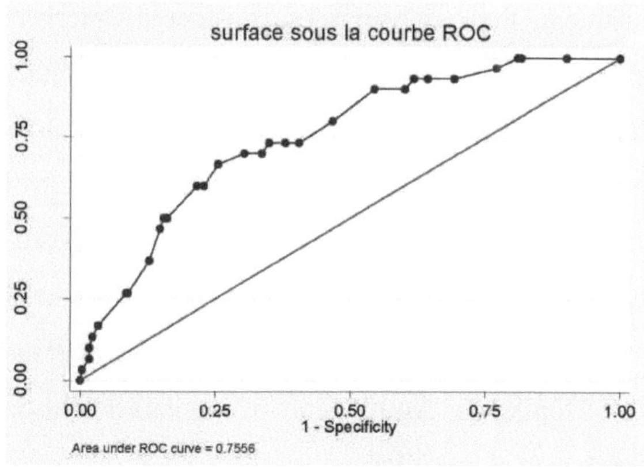

Figure 4: Goodness-of-fit test of the perinatal mortality model

With an area under the ROC curve of 76%, we conclude that the estimated model has good predictive power, with a specificity of 100% and a negative predictive value of 91%. This predicted model enabled us to correctly classify 91% of newborns.

II.3.3. Maternal characteristics and morbidity

Table XXIV shows the factors associated with maternal morbidity in cases of delivery on a scarred uterus.

Table XXIII: Factors associated with maternal morbidity and AUC

Features		Crude OR (IC95%)	P	Adjusted OR (IC95%)	P
Intergenerational interval (months)					
	-> 24 months	1		1	
-<	24 months	2,82 (1,34 - 5,94)	0,005	3,37(1,53 -7,41)	0,003
Website					
	-HASC	1		1	
	-HGRB	1,73(0,93 - 3,22)	0,081	1,29(0,62 - 2,70)	0,5
	-SENDWE	1,28(0,62 - 2,64)	0,5	1,20(0,54 - 2,65)	0,651
	-CUL	0,48(0,18 - 1,26)	0,127	0,33(0,11 -0,99)	0,049

After adjustment, the two variables considered, intergenital interval and delivery site, were significantly associated with maternal morbidity. An intergenital interval of less than 24 months (35.1%) was associated with a 3-fold greater risk of maternal morbidity in patients with scar uterus, compared with those with an interval of at least 24 months (16.1%); the difference observed was statistically significant. As for delivery site, patients attended at the Cliniques Universitaires de Lubumbashi (9.4%) were 3 times less likely to experience maternal morbidity than those attended at the Hôpital de l'Amitié Sino - Congolais in Kinshasa (17.9%), with a significant difference. (Table XXIV).

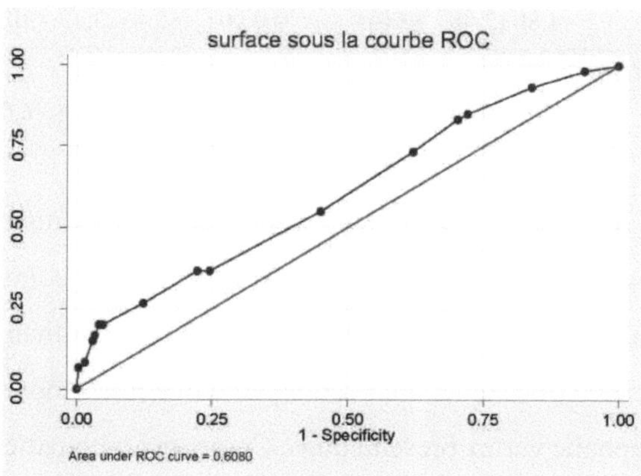

Figure 5: Goodness-of-fit test of the maternal morbidity model

As the area under the ROC curve of the estimated model is 61%, we can say that the estimated model has good predictive power, with a specificity of 100% and a negative predictive value of 82%. This model enabled us to classify 82% of patients correctly.

II.3.4. Factors associated with failure of the uterine test

Table XXIV: Factors associated with failure of the uterine test

Features	Crude OR (IC95%)	P	Adjusted OR (IC95%)	P
Age (years)				
-<20	2,64 (1,04 - 6,67)	0,041	3,32 (1,11 - 9,87)	0,031
-20 - 35	1		1	
->35	1,70 (1,10 - 2,64)	0,019	2,58 (0,89 - 2,80)	0,119
Parity				
-< 4	1		1	
-> 4	1,66 (1,10 - 2,51)	0,017	1,43 (0,82 - 2,52)	0,211
Water pocket				
-Rompue	4,76 (2,86 - 7,92)	< 0,001	3,95 (2,26 -6,90)	< 0,001
-Intact	1		1	
Presentation				
-Summit	1		1	

-Other	4,80 (2,88 - 8,00)	< 0,001	5,46 (3,13 - 10,95)	< 0,001
Uterine height (cm)				
-< 34	3,27 (1,62 - 6,59)	0,001	2,75 (1,26 - 6,00)	0,011
-> 34	1		1	

Table XXV shows that age, water sac status, uterine height and fetal presentation were explanatory factors in uterine test outcome. Patients under 20 years of age were 3 times more likely to fail a uterine test than those aged between 20 and 35. Presentations other than vertex were five times more likely to fail uterine testing than cephalic vertex presentations. Compared with patients admitted with an intact water sac, those admitted with a ruptured water sac were 4 times more likely to fail the uterine test. The risk of failure of the uterine test for patients with a uterine height exceeding 30 cm was 3 times higher than for parturients with a uterine height of less than 30 cm. The Hosmer Lemeshow test shows that the model achieves probabilities close to those observed.

Table XXV: Validity of the predicted model

Result obtained with the model	**Uterine test response observed**		**Total**
	Failure	***Success***	
Failure	132	43	175
Success	37	111	148
Total	**169**	**154**	**323**

Table XXVI shows that the predicted model correctly classifies 75.2% of uterine tests, with a sensitivity of 78.1%, a specificity of 72.1%, a positive predictive value of 75.4% and a negative predictive value of 75.0%.

Chapter 3

PREDICTIVE SCORE FOR OUTCOME OF UTERINE TEST OR PAUM SCORE

0. Introduction

The conclusions drawn from the previous chapters make it imperative to construct a predictive score for uterine test failure, based on a proper identification and analysis of the determinants of maternal-fetal outcome and uterine test. These determinants will need to be scored and their power determined. The score will be validated in a reliable experiment. The use of this predictive model in patients will improve quality in indications for the upper route, increase prophylactic caesarean section rates and optimize selection of patients for uterine testing. This should lead to a reduction in maternal-fetal morbidity and mortality associated with the management of delivery in a scarred uterus.

1. Methodological approach to score production

A total of 382 patients (17 of whom had benefited directly from an elective caesarean section) were included in the second part of our study, which focused on the determinants of maternal foetal outcome and uterine testing.

In this chapter, dedicated to the development of a predictive score for delivery in a scar uterus, the 17 patients who underwent an elective caesarean section were excluded from the analyses. Thus, only 365 patients undergoing spontaneous uterine testing (neither induced nor stimulated) were retained.

After constructing a third logistic regression model to identify factors associated with uterine test failure, only variables with a p-value < 0.05 and less likely to be subjective were introduced into the multivariate analysis. To reduce the likely bias on subjectivity in the information, certain parameters such as marital status, abortion history and delivery site were not introduced into the multivariate analysis. From this model, a score was constructed to predict uterine test failure in the four DRC hospital institutions selected for the study (Table XXVII), and given the acronym PAUM in reference to the initials of its constituent keywords, namely:

- Fetal presentation
- Maternal age
- Uterine height ;
- Membrane rupture.

Each modality of the variable was assigned a score according to its weight in the logistic regression model. The ROC curve was used to assess the score's ability to identify at-risk patients who are likely to experience uterine test failure. The threshold of the predictive score was determined on the basis of optimal sensitivity and specificity via the Youden index. All tests were performed at a threshold of a=0.05.

2. Predictive scoring

Table XXVI: Predictive score criteria

Score criteria	Score
Presentation	
-Occipital	1
-Other	4
Age (years)	
-< 20	3
-20 - 35	1
-> 35	2
Uterine height (cm)	
-< 34	1
-> 34	3
Membrane condition	
- Rompue	4
- Intact	1

Table XXVII clearly shows that, based on the Odds ratios provided by the logistic regression model, a score was created with a minimum and maximum of 4 and 16 respectively. The threshold obtained was 7, and was determined on the basis of optimal sensitivity and specificity using Youden's index. A total score greater than or equal to 7 indicated a risk of failure of the uterine test.

Figure 6: Goodness-of-fit test of the proposed model on uterine test outcome prediction

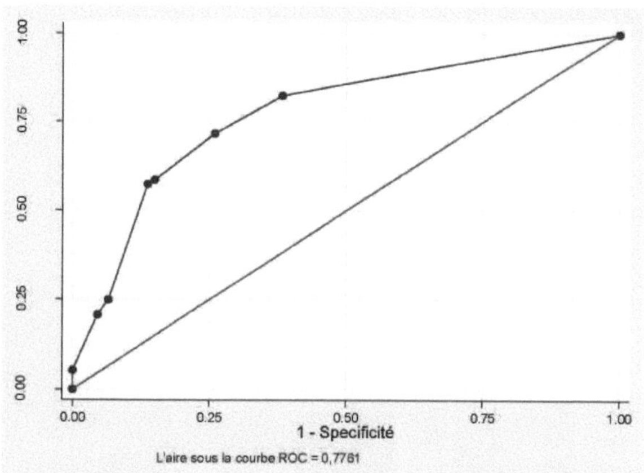

The score for predicting scar uterus deliveries enables 72.7% of uterine tests to be correctly classified, with a sensitivity of 71.6%, a specificity of 74.0%, a positive predictive value of 75.1% and a negative predictive value of 70.4%.

3. Internal validation of the predictive score

Table XXVII: Validity of the prediction score of the proposed model

Prediction score for AUC	Uterine test response observed *Failure*	*Success*	Total
> 7	121	40	161
< 7	48	114	162
Total	**169**	**154**	**323**

Of the 323 patients entered in the logistic regression model to predict uterine test, 235 (121 + 114), or 73%, were correctly classified with the proposed score. This score has a sensitivity of 72%, a specificity of 74%, a positive predictive value of 75, % and a negative predictive value of 70%.

Chapter 4

DISCUSSION

In this chapter, we discuss the results of our study, try to explain them and, where possible, compare them with the scientific literature.

This discussion will first address the methodological limitations of the study, before focusing on the results themselves.

IV.1 Methodological discussion

Our research is prospective, multicentric, cross-sectional and analytical. As we know, a cross-sectional study does not allow for trend analysis, which would have been a remarkable added value.

Although not representative of all maternity units in the DRC, the 4 study sites were not randomly selected, which could suggest a selection bias. It would have been desirable to have at least one study site in the east of the DRC in order to cover the whole country. However, this was not possible, mainly due to operational constraints. To simplify recruitment procedures, as mentioned above, we only included patients from the four maternity units that care for a large number of patients with scarred uteruses, and which attract patients from different communes in the towns concerned. These four maternity hospitals and the population they serve are probably no different from those not included in the study. Thus, the results of this study can reasonably be reported for the country as a whole, assuming that there are no major biotypic differences between patients in Kinshasa, Mbuji - Mayi and Lubumbashi, on the one hand, and those in the rest of the DRC, on the other.

Some information, such as abortion history, marital status, parity and number of previous caesarean sections, was reported to us by the patients. The technique used to collect this data exposed us to the risk of misclassification (information bias). The classification errors (lack of internal validity) that could occur if questions were poorly formulated in the questionnaire (data collection form) would have reduced the ability to highlight the real effect of risk factors on the phenomenon studied by underestimating the odds ratio (directional bias towards unity or dilution of the effect). The care taken in designing and validating the questionnaire, as well as the very regular monitoring of the interviewers in the field, had made it possible to minimize such errors.

As for possible confounding factors, in the design of this research, we restricted participation in the study to pregnant women with 1 or 2 previous caesarean sections. We then used multivariate analyses, and no confounding was found after adjustment of the estimated models. This did not prevent the survival of residual confounding, as not all variables thought to explain the outcome of the uterine test were introduced into the model. This residual confusion could, moreover, result from the way we categorized certain continuous variables such as the age and parity of the pregnant bitch.

To ensure that the results of our study are highly accurate, we used a sufficiently large sample size, with acceptable statistical power; the accuracy of the results depending on the sample size, the variability of the parameters studied (95% CI of frequency and effect measures) and the absence or presence of random errors, including the three main sampling sources of measurement, classification and individual biological variation.

Despite the above-mentioned limitations, this study has the merit of being the first in the Democratic Republic of Congo to propose a score for predicting the outcome of a uterine test, which we call **the PAUM SCORE**.

IV .2. Frequency of delivery on scar uterus

Since 2005, the WHO has published annual global health statistics showing the evolution of caesarean section rates worldwide.

Caesarean section surgery, initially considered a life-saving procedure, has become a safety practice, with scar uterus and dystocia as its two main indications

[12]. Since the main cause of scar uterus is a previous caesarean section, it is important to describe the evolution of caesarean section rates, which determine the subsequent frequency of AUC. The increase in caesarean section rates over the past 20 years is a widely shared phenomenon in both developed and developing countries. Indeed, in most developed countries, this rate is well above 15% (the threshold long defined as optimal by the WHO), and around 5 to 7% in developing countries (the interval long defined as minimal by the WHO). The inevitable consequence of the trend in Caesarean section rates is that the prevalence of scar uterus has risen from 7% to 14% in most countries, both in Africa and worldwide [3].

What's more, Smith et al [3] reported in 2005 that the inflationary trend in caesarean section rates has led proportionately to an increase in the frequency of AUC, with enormous variation from one country to another, from one city to another, and within the same setting, from one hospital institution to another.

The frequency of scar uterus deliveries during this study period was 6.53%. In France, between 1995 and 2010, the prevalence of scar uteri increased from 8% to 11%, according to ACOG data reported in 2010 [10]. This result is close to the African data reported in Yaoundé (Cameroon) in 2004 (4.7%) and Dar-Es-Salaam (Tanzania) (7.7%) [13]. On the other hand, it is lower than the frequencies of 8.4% and 9% described respectively at the Cliniques Universitaires de Kinshasa in 2013 [14] and in Kigali in 2005 (Rwanda) and Kampala (Uganda) in 2006 [13]. In almost 30 years, we note that the frequency of scar uterus deliveries has tripled, rising from 2.43% in 1983 to 8.45% in 2010 at the Cliniques Universitaires de Kinshasa [14,19]. This inflation in the rate of scar-uterine deliveries is proportional to the evolution of the caesarean section rate, which increased almost tenfold over the same period, from 3.69% in 1983 to 30.6% in 2010 [14]. This could be explained, on the one hand, by the fact that the hospitals included in our study are either secondary or tertiary level, and on the other hand, some of them are, in their respective provinces, structures at the top of the health pyramid, whose maternity units give priority to high-risk deliveries. However, the methodology used could have an underestimating effect, as the present study only considered scar uteri secondary to caesarean section, to the detriment of non-obstetric scars. The frequency could also be affected by the exclusion from the outset of multi-catric uteri (>2), pregnancies under 34 weeks' gestation with multiple contents, scar uteri with absolute contraindications to vaginal delivery, and scar uteri with fetal death in utero.

V V.3 Morbi - maternal mortality

In our series, 79 cases (20.68%) presented at least one complication, dominated by haemorrhage (41.77%) and post-partum endometritis (34.18%). Uterine rupture was diagnosed in 6 cases (7.59%), with no significant difference between the sites studied. Delivery haemorrhage was more frequent in vaginal delivery (HGRB: 14.06%) than in the groups marked by upper-route delivery, but with no significant statistical difference, suggesting that the primary cause was likely to be the uterine atony common to irrational disproportionate trials of the vaginal route, rather than uterine scarring. Haemorrhagic complications are recognized as the leading cause of obstetric mortality in developing countries [20,21]. As far as infectious pathologies are concerned, post-partum endometritis, unfortunately frequent in the literature with a rate varying between 1.9% and 30% [22], is the most dreaded complication, as it weakens the uterine scar and exposes the patient to subsequent uterine rupture. In our study, the high rates of post-partum endometritis could be explained by the equally high frequency of low socio-economic status and precarious surgical environment, early opening of membranes and systematic manual revision of the uterine cavity after delivery to exclude disunion of the old scar, which is common practice notably at the BIMPEBA General Reference Hospital in Mbuji - Mayi, in Lubumbashi at SENDWE and at the Cliniques Universitaires de Lubumbashi.

Finally, the real problem posed by gravid scar uteri is the fear of uterine rupture, which justifies obstetrical attitudes that are as varied as they are frustrating.

Our study reports a uterine rupture rate of 1.57%, statistically independent of the site considered. The same applies to maternal mortality (1.31%), irrespective of the mode of delivery. These rates, which are comparable to those of other authors on the continent, and even in developed countries [13, 14, 17, 19, 22, 23], reassure us of the good quality of the uterine scar in Caesarean sections performed in a precarious environment, and of the need to pay particular attention to the parturition of a scarred uterus, with a view to contraindicating its continuation, if necessary.

VI .4. Morbi - perinatal mortality

The APGAR score at five minutes shows a higher rate of neonatal depression at the Hôpital de l'Amitié Sino - Congolais in Kinshasa (57.8%) and at the Cliniques Universitaires in Lubumbashi (50.60%) than at the Hôpital SENDWE in Lubumbashi (31.2%) and at the Hôpital Général de Référence in Lubumbashi.

BIMPEBA in Mbuji - Mayi (16.0%), contrasting paradoxically with a lower perinatal mortality rate in the former group (5.11%) than in the latter (10.68%), with a statistically significant difference (p=0.04). Could this be due to a flaw in the assessment of the APGAR score, or to shortcomings in neonatal resuscitation? The question arises in view of the fact that both skills require appropriate training, expertise and infrastructure, which are more readily available in the city and in university training facilities than on the outskirts of the city. Whatever the reasons, the perinatal morbidity and mortality rates found in this study are comparable to those reported in the African literature [7, 8, 14, 17], and suggest that efforts should be made to improve perinatal management in cases of parturition in a scarred uterus (intrapartum electronic monitoring, qualified neonatal assistance).

VII 5. Delivery procedures

The disparity in results reported in the literature is due, among other reasons, to differing medical conditions and the absence of a homogeneous attitude among obstetricians when faced with delivery on a scarred uterus [12]. Some authors authorize uterine testing in 27.8% of cases, with success rates ranging from 45 to 92.5% [12]. In our study, almost half the patients delivered vaginally, irrespective of the geographical location of the hospital. The high rate of uterine testing in the three maternity hospitals in Kinshasa (Hôpital de l'Amitié Sino - Congolais) and Lubumbashi (Cliniques Universitaires and SENDWE) may be attributable to the rigorous selection of cases submitted to uterine testing in order to maximize the chances of success, since the rate of vaginal deliveries after caesarean section depends on the quality of patient selection. In fact, it has been reported that complications of scar uterus occur mainly with uterine testing [13]. The high rate observed at the BIMPEBA General Referral Hospital in Mbuji - Mayi, in an environment where the obstetrical technical platform and qualified personnel are sorely lacking, should make us reflect on the objectives we are really pursuing when choosing the delivery route. In short, the relatively low rate of vaginal deliveries is by no means synonymous with a "low rate of attempted vaginal deliveries", as failures have certainly been punished by Caesarean section. Between the fear of complications for some practitioners and recklessness for others, there could be, at different rates depending on the site, on the one hand many abusive caesarean sections and, on the other, missed opportunities for caesarean section, given the amount of fetomaternal morbidity involved.

VIII . Determinants of uterine test failure

The factors associated with failure of the uterine test provide the obstetrician with early information on the possibilities of natural childbirth.

The failure rate of uterine testing varies in the literature. It ranges from 13 to 51% [15, 57]. The 67 studies in the meta-analysis by Guise et al (14 prospective and 53 retrospective) [57] show that the success rate of uterine testing was 74% (95% CI [75, 36], n =368,304), with significant heterogeneity (I^2 >98%), without any explanatory factors being found for this difference (year of study, country of origin of the study, term of delivery and type of study).

Our study identified four explanatory factors for uterine test failure, which were used to define the score's acronym **PAUM**, namely:

- Fetal presentation and
- Maternal age ;
- Uterine height ;
- Premature rupture of membranes.

1. Maternal age and uterine test failure

The aim of this discussion is to determine whether, in our environment, there is a maternal age threshold above or below which, due to a low success rate for uterine testing and/or a high maternal-perinatal complication rate, a caesarean section would be preferable to TAVB on a scarred uterus.

With a non-identical mean in the four maternity units included in the study (p = 0.017), patients in our series had a mean age of 31.28 ±7.38 years. In bivariate analysis, the highest proportion of perinatal morbidity was recorded among patients aged over 35 (OR: 4.33; IC95%: 1.23 - 15.25; p= 0.022). And after adjustment with logistic regression, maternal age was statistically associated with perinatal morbidity. As one of the explanatory factors for uterine test outcome, and compared with age 20 to 35, age under 20 was 3 times more likely to experience uterine test failure.

The long-term obstetrical consequences of elective caesarean section in elderly patients are not the same as in younger patients, since the possibilities of future pregnancies are less important in this sub-population. Several authors agree that AUC rates increase directly with age: lower for patients under twenty and higher for those over forty [43].

In 2002, the study by Bujold et al (n=2493) [43] of patients with no previous natural delivery indicated that uterine rupture success rates were 71.9%, 70.7% and 65.1% (p=0.06) respectively for patients under 30, 30-35 and over 35 years of age, and 91.5%, 91.1% and 82.9% (p=0.005) for patients with a previous natural delivery. Uterine rupture rates did not differ between these age groups: 2.0%, 1.1% and 1.4% (p=0.404) for patients with no previous history of vaginal delivery, and 0.0%, 0.3% and 0.9% for those with previous vaginal deliveries. In 2003, on the other hand, a study by Shipp et al [29] involving over 3,000 patients reported that maternal age over 30 years increased the risk of uterine rupture by a factor of 3. This difference persisted even after adjustment for birth weight, interval between caesarean section and subsequent delivery, induction of labour and use of oxytocin.

Two studies [47, 58] investigated the effect of maternal age on the risk of uterine rupture and on the success rate of uterine testing. They concluded that increasing maternal age reduced the possibility of natural delivery. This finding is not specific to patients with scarred uteri, as it has also been described in patients with unscarred uteri [84].

Eight cohort studies reported in uni or multivariate analysis an association between maternal age and the success rate of uterine testing. Five of these studies found a higher success rate among patients under 40 years of age [10, 43], while the other three found no significant difference in the success rate of uterine testing as a function of maternal age [13, 59].

In any case, the literature does not provide sufficient evidence to determine a maternal age threshold above which an elective caesarean section is preferable to uterine testing, in the case of UA. However, the patient's obstetrical future is a factor to be taken into account when informing and deciding on the mode of delivery for these patients.

Although it would be excessive to conclude that patient age alone would be associated with the success and/or failure of uterine testing, several authors agree on two main facts: that age alone has no influence on uterine scar quality except through parity, and that there is a causal relationship between increasing age and maternal-perinatal morbidity [10, 43, 60]

2. Uterine height and failure of the uterine test

In our series, patients with a scar uterus whose uterine height was greater than 34 cm were significantly associated with the risk of failure during uterine testing (OR: 2.73; CI95%: 1.13 - 6.57).

As fetal weight is an antenatal parameter in the methodology used, it was excluded from the logistic regression model for two main reasons: firstly, it is naturally associated with uterine height (subjective reliability because it is operator-dependent), which can lead to model instability due to collinearity; secondly, the prediction of failure or success of the uterine test with regard to the weight parameter of the newborn assumes that the latter has already been born (unless we refer, while assuming its limitations, to ultrasound weight). This is why we have a proxy variable, in this case uterine height, which also indirectly measures fetal weight, while offering a practical and economic advantage (ultrasound is not available to everyone). As multiple pregnancies are excluded from our study, and no cases of hydramnios have been reported, we will only deal with aspects related to fetal macrosomia.

Some authors recommend prophylactic caesarean section in the face of uterine overdistension, which they consider to be a formal contraindication to uterine testing [43, 60]. Others, on the other hand, have tried to demonstrate, without determining the cause, that uterine overdistension cannot contraindicate vaginal delivery on a scarred uterus [25].

The probability of vaginal delivery in a scar uterus is directly related to fetal weight [39].

The occurrence of fetal macrosomia in a previously caesareanized patient is a frequent occurrence, accounting for around 16% of scar-uterine deliveries. In the literature, the success rate of uterine testing in patients who have given birth to macrosomia varies between 40% and 92%, the average noted in a review of the literature compiling 807 cases [61, 62] being 69%.

Flamm [63] reports a success rate of 78% for the group with a birth weight < 4,000 g, 58% for the group with a birth weight between 4,000 and 4,499 g, and only 43% if the birth weight is greater than 4,500 g. Flamm [63] also notes that the rate of vaginal delivery of macrosomia in previously caesareanized patients is statistically significantly lower (90% *vs.* 55%), compared with the test of labour in a non-scarred uterus.

The risk of uterine rupture during uterine testing in cases of fetal macrosomia is estimated at 0.3% in Flamm's series [63] of 301 cases, and 0.7% in Phelan's series [39] of 140 cases. This risk seems similar to that observed in cases of normal fetal weight (<4,000 g). The risk of uterine dehiscence was around 0.7% in the Flamm series [63] and 2.1% for Phelan [39]. This risk is no different from that for fetal weights under 4,000 g.

In the case of fetal macrosomia, TAVB presents a major risk of shoulder dystocia, which exposes the patient to the risk of obstetrical trauma, including brachial plexus palsy [61]. However, the majority of authors consider that in the absence of other risk factors, in particular maternal diabetes, a suspicion of fetal macrosomia does not justify the systematic practice of Caesarean section, especially as current techniques for estimating fetal weight are not sufficiently reliable [39].

Secondary caesarean section after failure of the uterine test is associated with greater maternal morbidity, particularly serious complications [64]. A thorough clinical, and sometimes para-clinical, assessment of obstetric conditions prior to uterine testing is therefore of paramount importance, as it helps to exclude poor feto-pelvic confrontations and avoid uterine testing that is doomed to failure due to potential complications. Once the uterine test has been accepted, active management of labor, under strict supervision by a trained obstetric team, is essential. It is essential to draw up a partogram in order to detect and treat any abnormalities in labor in good time. Stagnation of dilatation in the active phase of labor beyond 2 hours after correction of dynamic abnormalities, as well as failure to engage the fetal head after one hour of full dilatation, should lead to interruption of the uterine test and Caesarean section.

3. Premature rupture of the membranes and failure of the uterine test

Numerous studies have looked at obstetric factors in labor to predict uterine test success. Three prospective studies and one case-control study showed that the success rate of uterine testing increased with cervical dilatation at admission or at the time of rupture of membranes. The two studies that looked at cervical effacement showed that the increase in the success rate of uterine testing was related to the percentage of cervical effacement, by a factor of two to six as the BISHOP score in the labour room increased [4].

Some authors have suggested a relative risk of hyperkinetic labour in early labour, as prostaglandin levels in amniotic fluid are always higher than maternal levels, at 24 to 85 pg for PGE and 5 to 10 pg for PGF [65]. Amniotic fluid contains the prostaglandins PGE2 and PGF2, which increase the number of uterine receptors for oxytocics and potentiate their uterotonic effect [4, 22, 66, 67].

As with a scar-free uterus, the risk of cord procidence increases with premature rupture of membranes [66].

In our series, a ruptured water sac (OR: 3.95; CI95% :2.26 - 6.90) was statistically associated with uterine test failure. Premature rupture of the membranes in the case of pathologies concomitant with pregnancy was reported in 11% of patients, meaning that almost one in three patients (34%) was practically admitted with a ruptured water bag. This proportion was higher at the HGRB and exceeded 40% at the two Lubumbashi hospitals. On the other hand, there were more vaginal deliveries among patients admitted with a ruptured water bag, four times more than among those admitted with an intact bag (OR: 3.94; IC95%: 2.44 - 6.37). In bivariate analysis, the condition of the water bag on admission was statistically associated with perinatal morbidity. Indeed, 43% of cases of perinatal morbidity were recorded in patients admitted with a ruptured water bag, compared with only 29% in patients admitted with an intact water bag (p=0.012). In addition, 63% of perinatal mortality cases were recorded in patients admitted with a ruptured water bag, compared with only 37% in patients admitted with an intact water bag (p=0.002). Also, in multivariate analysis, patients with early rupture of membranes were 4 times more likely to have their child die during the perinatal period (OR: 3.82; 95% CI: 1.67 - 8.71; p=0.001). After adjustment with logistic regression, ruptured water on admission was significantly associated with perinatal morbidity and mortality.

4. Presentation and failure of the uterine test

Our discussion will focus on deflexed presentations (bregma and face), posterior varieties of vertex and breech presentation. Transverse and forehead presentations, which are frankly dystocic, have been excluded from our study.

In the human species, cephalo-pelvic confrontation forces the fetal head to flex for delivery in order to reduce its anteroposterior diameter. In less than 1% of cases, this mechanism does not occur, leaving instead a more or less significant deflection of the head. This defines deflected cephalic presentations. These presentations are characterized by long labor and complex obstetrical mechanics. Posterior varieties of vertex presentation appear classically less eutocile than anterior varieties, with a less favourable obstetrical and fetal prognosis [67].

When a scarred uterus is associated with a presentation other than well-flexed cephalic, the commonly adopted attitude is to perform a systematic iterative caesarean section [68]. However, this attitude is not accepted by some authors, who report that uterine testing in breech presentation gives good results, with low complication rates [69]. Vaginal delivery of a breech fetus poses a risk of uterine rupture during extraction. Fearing this risk in a scarred uterus, some authors opt for a systematic iterative caesarean section in the presence of a scarred uterus and breech presentation [4, 33]. This contrasts with other authors who report a low complication rate when performing a uterine test on a breech presentation [70].

In our series, patients with a presentation other than occipital cephalic (OR: 5.46; 95% CI: 3.13 - 10.95) were at risk of failure during uterine testing. This suggests a possible link with the genesis of dystocic presentations, the etiologies of which differ for each of them.

Consequently, the detection of a dystocic presentation during the 3rd trimester of gestation requires more frequent consultations and an etiological investigation of the presentation before concluding that it is idiopathic in origin.

IV.7. AUC prediction score

The aim of predictive scores is to assess the probability of success of the uterine test [71], on the one hand, and of failure of the same test on the other [72].

In their retrospective study of 10828 scar uteri, Bensaid et al [70] developed an internally validated predictive score for successful uterine testing. Only three factors were associated with successful uterine testing (absence of recurrent cause of CS, absence of history of fetal macrosomia and absence of maternal anemia). This score establishes a rating of 1 (one) when the factor was absent and another of 0 (zero) when it was present.

Other authors have attempted to establish an antenatal score predictive of uterine test failure in a case-control study of 336 subjects. This study predicted a uterine test failure rate in 63% of cases, although some other authors question the reliability of this score [74, 75].

In their series, Flamm et al [47] studied a prospective cohort of 5000 patients, and selected five factors to predict the success rate of the uterine test (maternal age, history of AVB, indication for previous CS, vaginal touch on admission, dilatation and degree of cervical effacement). A positive correlation was found between the success rate of the uterine test and the calculated score, ranging from 49.1% for scores 0 - 2 to 94.9% for scores 8 - 10.

In our series, two types of explanatory factors for uterine test failure were selected. The first was the sociodemographic factor (maternal age) and the second three obstetrical factors (uterine height, fetal presentation and premature rupture of membranes).

The score we defined to predict uterine test failure was based on these four elements: maternal age, status of the water sac on admission, uterine height and fetal presentation. With a minimum score of 4, a maximum score of 16 and a cut-off point of 7, a total score of 7 or more indicates a risk of uterine test failure.

Most of the scores reported were based on small numbers, retrospective cohorts or cohorts that were too old, with outdated medical practices, which introduces numerous biases.

Our score validated a fairly robust methodology (prospective study, logistic regression, internal validation) whose area under the ROC curve of 74% made its reliability acceptable.

CONCLUSION

In undertaking this work, we were motivated by the desire to make a contribution to the prevention and/or minimization of the risk of maternal morbidity and mortality in the event of parturition on a scar uterus in a resource-limited obstetrical environment. The present study therefore aims to contribute to the reduction of maternal and perinatal morbidity and mortality through the rational management of scar uterus deliveries in low-resource hospital settings.

To achieve this, we conducted a prospective, multicenter, cross-sectional and analytical study of patients with scarred uteri in four different hospital institutions in the Democratic Republic of Congo, namely:

1. Hôpital de l'Amitié Sino - Congolaise (HASC), Kinshasa
2. BIMPEBA General Reference Hospital (HGRB) in Mbuji - Mayi
3. Lubumbashi University Clinics
4. SENDWE Hospital, Lubumbashi

This study enabled us to identify 4 determinants of maternal-fetal outcome and uterine challenge, and maternal and neonatal morbidity and mortality, which define the PAUM score for predicting uterine challenge failure.

The use of this predictive score in patients should result in improved quality in indications for the upper approach, higher rates of prophylactic caesarean sections, and better selection of patients undergoing uterine testing. We are convinced that all these effects will contribute to a reduction in maternal-fetal morbidity associated with the management of delivery in scarred uteri.

We therefore recommend :

Obstetricians, general practitioners and obstetricians: to use this score before making any decision on the choice of route for delivery in a scar uterus;

To the DRC's hospital institutions, the privileged beneficiaries of this score: to hold training sessions for obstetricians, general practitioners and midwives. We believe that raising awareness at grassroots level is the best way to ensure that our modest contribution has a definite multiplier effect;

To the Ministry of Public Health: to adopt the use of this score in the national reproductive health policy and to popularize, with its **Partners**, its experimentation and use on a national scale;

The Ministry of Higher Education and Universities, through its specialized programs: to give a new direction to the obstetrics course given in the various medical faculties, based on this score predicting the outcome of the uterine test.

BIBLIOGRAPHY

1. **Durnwald C, Mercer B.** *Vaginal birth after cesarean delivery: predicting success, risks of failure.* J Matern Fetal Neonatal Med. 2004 Jun; 15(6): 388-93.
2. **Aboulfalah A, Abbassi H, El karroumi M, Morsad F, Samouh N.** *Delivery of large baby on scar uterus: the place of uterine testing about 355 cases.* J. Gynecol. Obstet. Biol. Reprod.2000 ;29 : 409-413.
3. **Smith GCS, White IR, Pell JP, Dobbie R.** *Predicting cesarean section and uterine rupture among women attemping vaginal birth after prior cesarean section.* Plos. Med.2005; 2.
4. **Haumonte JB, Raylet M, Sabiani L, Francke O, Bretelle F, Boubli L.** *What factors influence the route of delivery in case of attempted vaginal delivery on scar uterus? J* Gynecol Obstet Biol Reprod, 2012.13.
5. **Acog Committee Opinion.** *Induction of labor for vaginal birth after caesarean delivery.* Int, J. Gynecol. Obstet.2002; 77: 303-304.
6. **Organization For Economic Cooperation And Developpement.** Health Data. Accessed on 04/07/2012: http://wwwoecdorg/health/healthdata
   Médecine d'Afrique Noire. 2006 ;5305 : 293-298
7. **Adjahoto E O, Ekoevi DK, Hodonou K.** *Predictive factors for the outcome of uterine testing in an under-equipped setting.* J. Gynecol. Obstet. Biol. Reprod.2001 ;30 : 174-179.
8. **Kizonde K, Kinekinda X, Kimbala J, Kamwenyi K.** *Caesarean section in the African environment. Exemple de la maternité centrale Sendwe de Lubumbashi - R.D. Congo.* Médecine d'Afrique Noire, 2006; 5305: 293 - 298.
9. **Fitzpatrick KE, Kurinczuk JJ, Alfirevic Z, Spark P, Brocklehurst P, Knight M**. *Uterine rupture by intended mode of delivery in the UK: a national case - control study.* PLoS Med. 2012; 9: e1 001184.

10. **American College Of Obstetricians And Gynaecologists**. *Mode of term single breech delivery: ACOG committee opinion number 265.* J. Obstet. Gynecol.2001; 98: 189-190.
11. **Appleton B, Targett C, Rasmussen M, Readman E, Sale F.** *Vaginal birth after Caesarean section: an Australian multicentre study*. Aust N Z J Obstet Gynaecol, 2000; vol. 40, p. 87-91.
12. **Cassignol C, Rudigoz CR**. *Pregnancy and scar uterus*. E.M.C., 2003; 5-016-D-20.
13. **Zelop CM, Shipp TD, Cohen A, Repke JT, Lieberman E**. *Trial of labor after 40 weeks 'gestation in women with prior cesarean. Obstet Gynecol.*2001; 97:391-3.
14. **Boffendakini JR, Rahma RT, Lokomba BV.** *Delivery on scarred uterus at Cliniques Universitaires de Kinshasa, Annales Africaines de Médecine.* 2013; volume 6, number3; 1430 - 1437.
15. **Blondel B, Lelong N, Kermarrec M, Goffinet F.** *Trends in perinatal health in France between 1995 and 2010: results from the national perinatal surveys.* J Gynecol Obstet Biol Reprod (Paris). 2012; 41:151-66.
16. **American College Of Obstetricians And Gynecologists.** *Vaginal birth after previous cesarean delivery, clinical management guidelines for Obstetrician-Gynecologists*. ACOG Pract Bull. 1998; 54 : 1-10.
17. **Society of Obstetricians, Gynaecologists of Canada, SOGC.** *Clinical Practice Guidelines for vaginal birth after previous caesarean birth, Number 155 (Replaces guideline Number 147).* February Int J Gynaecol Obstet. 2005; 89 : 319-331.
18. **Royal College of Obstetricians and Gynaecologists.** *Birth after previous caesarean section. Green Top Guideline*. 2005; February No 45.
19. **Tshilombo KM, Mputu L, Nguma M, Wolomby M, Tozin R, Yanga K.** *Delivery in the previously cesareanized Zairean pregnant woman*. J Gynecol Obstet.1991; 20: 568 - 574.

20. **Nkunzumwami E**. *les enjeux sociopolitiques et économiques en république democratique du congo (rdc).* harmattan, Paris, ed. 2011, 56-89.

21. **Pridjian G**. *Labor after prior cesarean section*, Clin Obstet Gynecol *1992*; 35, 3: 445-456.

22. **Papiernick E, Cabrol D, Pons JC.** *Obstétrique.* Flammarion, Paris, 1ère éd.1998**;** 1191-1204.

23. **Cosson M, Dufon P, Nayama M, Vinatier D, Monnier JC.** *Obstetrical prognosis of scar uteri: A propos de 641 cas.* J Gynecol Obstet Biol Reprod. 1995; 24: 434-439.

24. **Sanchez-Ramos L, Gaudier FL, Kaunitz AM**. *Cervical ripening and labor induction after previous Cesarean delivery.* Clin Obstet Gynecol 2000; vol. 43, p. 513-23.

25. **Haddad S, Maria B.** *L'accouchement sur utérus cicatriciel à propos de 150 cas. Rev. Fr, Gynécol. Obstet. 1994 ; 89, 12, 606-612.*

26. **Demianczuk N, Hunter D, Tylor D**. *Trial labor after previous cesarean section: prognoses indicators of outcome*. Am J Obstet Gynecol1982; 142, 640-642.

27. **Lehmann M, Hedelin G, Sorgue C, Gollner GL, Grall C, Chami.** *Factors predictive of route of delivery in women with scar uterus.* J. Gynecol Obstet Biol Reprod 1999; 28: 358-368.

28. **Wasef WRK.** *An audit of trial of labour after previous caesarean sections.* J Obstet Gynaecol 2000; 20 (4): 380- 381.

29. **Shipp TD, Zelop C, Cohen A, Repke JT, Lieberman E.** *Post cesarean delivery fever and uterine rupture in a subsequent trial of labor.* Obstet. Gynecol. 2003; 101 (1): 136-139.

30. **Eng JJ, Sangla N, Tanoh L, Hocke G.** *Triggering on scar uterus.* Rev Fr Gynecol Obstét 1992; **87**, 4: 188-190.

31. **Bujold E, Mehta SH, Bujold C, Gauthier RJ.** *Interdelivery interval and uterine rupture. Am J Obstet Gynecol* 2002; 187: 1199-1202.

32. **Granovsky-Grisaru S, Shaya M, Diamant YZ.** *The management of labor in women with more than one uterine scar: Is a repeat cesarean section really the only "safe" option? J Perinat Med 1994*; 22: 13-7.
33. **Diallo FB, Diallo MS, Bangoura S, Diallo AB, Camara Y.** *Uterine rupture at the Niamey central referral maternity hospital.* Médecine Afrique Noire 1998, 45 (5): 310-315.
34. **Chattopadhay SK, Sherbeeni MM, Anokute CC**. *Planned vaginal delivery after two previous Cesarean sections.* Br J Obstet Gynecol 1994 vol 101, p. 498-500.
35. **Hamet Tidjani A, Gallais A, Garba M**. *L'accouchement sur utérus cicatriciel au niger: a propos de 590 cas.* Médecine d'Afrique Noire. 2001 ; 48 (2).
36. **Hammoud A, Hendler I, Gauthier R J, Berman S, Sansregret A, Bujolde.** *The effect of gestational age on trial of labor after cesarean section.* J Matern Fetal Neonatal Med.2004; 15:202-6.
37. **Ruiz- Velasco V, Beltran FR, Bejarano OT**. Delivery after caesarean section: morbimortality. *J Gynecol Obstet Biol Reprod.*1973 ;*2*: 673684.
38. **Huang WH, Nakashima DK, Rumney PJ, Keegan KA, Chan K.** *Interdelivery interval and the success of vaginal birth after cesarean delivery.* Obstet. Gynecol, 2002; 99 (1) : 41-44.
39. **Phelan JP, Eglinton GS, Horenstein JM, Clark SL, Yeh Sze-Ya.** *Previous cesarean birth: trial of labor in women with macrosomic infants*. J Reprod Med; 1984. 29: 36-40.
40. **Myles TD, Santolaya-Fargas J.** *Vaginal birth after cesarean delivery: predictors of success or failure.* Obstet Gynecol 2002; 99 (4) suppl: 5556.
41. **Lansac J, Magnin G**. *Obstétrique* . 4th edition. Paris : Masson. 2008.
42. **Akotionga M, Lankoande J, Gue M J, Kone B.** *Uterine ruptures at the CHN-YO maternity hospital.* Médecine Afrique Noire, 1998, 45 (8-9): 508-510.

43. **Bujold E, Mehta SH, Bujold C, Gauthier RJ.** *Interdelivery interval and uterine rupture.* Am. J. Obstet. Gynecol.2002; 187: 1199-1202.

44. **Bromley B, Pitcher BL, Klapholz H, Lichter E, Benacerral BR.** *Sonographicappearanceofuterine scardehiscence* . Int.J.Gynecol.Obstet.1995; 51: 53-56.

45. **Michaels WH, Thompson HO, Boutt A, Schreiber RF, Michaels SL.** *Ultrasound diagnosis of defects in the scarred lower uterine segment during pregnancy.* Obstet.Gynecol.1998; 1: 112-120.

46. **Martel MJ, MacKinnon CJ.** *Clinical Practice Obstetrics Committee, Society of Obstetricians and Gynaecologists of Canada. Guidelines for vaginal birth after previous Caesarean birth.* J Obstet Gynaecol Can. 2005 Feb; 27(2):164-88.

47. **Flamm BL, Newman LA, Thomas ST, Fallon D, Yoshida MM.** *Vaginal Birth after cesarean delivery: results of a 5 year multicenter collaborative study.* Obstet gynecol, 1990; 76:750-4.

48. **Garg VK, Ekuma-Nkama EN.** *Vaginal birth following caesarean deliveries: Are the risks exaggerated.* Ann Saud Med 2004 ; 24 (4): 276279.

49. **Esposito MA, Menihan CA, Malee MP.** *Association of inter pregnancy interval with uterine scar failure in labor: A case control study.* Am J Obstet Gynecol 2000, 183 (5).

50. **Khalek N, Blackwell S, Hendler I, Berman S, Gauthier R, Bujold E.** *Obstetric outcomes in women with two prior cesarean deliveries undergoing a trial of labor.* Am. J. Obstet. Gynecol.2003; 189 (6) : s125.

51. **Dicle O.** *Magnetic resonance imaging evaluation of incision healing after caesarean sections.* Eur. Radiol.1997; 7 : 31-34.

52. **Cahill A, Stamilio DM, Pare E, Peipert JP, Stevens EJ.** *Vaginal birth after cesarean (VBAC) attempt in twin pregnancies: is it safe?* Am J Obstet Gynecol, 2005; 193 (suppl.1), 1050-1055.

53. **Kraiem J, Ben Brahim Y, Chaabane K, Sarraj N, Chiha N, Falfoula A.**

Indicators for successful vaginary delivery after cesarean section: a proposal of a predictive score. Tunis Med, 2006, janvier; 84(1): 16-20.

54. **Kieser KE, Baskett TF**. *A 10-year population-based study of uterine rupture. Am J ObstetGynecol.*2002; vol. 100, p. 749-53.
55. **Adama D, Zekiba T, Ouédraogo J L, Oumarou T, Moussa B.** *Outcome of scar uterus deliveries in a university hospital in Burkina.* The Pan African Medical Journal. 2012; 12 : 95.
56. **Agency for Healthcare Research and Quality**. *Vaginal birth after cesarean: new insights.* AHRQ Publication N°.10-E003 2010.
57. **Picaud A, Nlome-Nze AR, Ogowet N, Engongah T, Ella-Ekogha A.** *Delivery of scar uteri: A propos de 606 cas pour 62193 accouchements*. Rev Fr, Gynecol Obstet1990; 85, (6): 387-392.
58. **Mercer BM, Gilbert S, Landon MB, Spong CY, Leveno KJ, Rou DJ.** *National Institute of Child Health and Human Development Maternal- Fetal Medicine Units Network. Labor outcomes with increasing number of prior vaginal births after cesarean delivery*. Obstet Gynecol.2008; 111:285-91
59. **Landon MB, Leindecker S, Spong CY, Bloom S, Varner MW, Moawad AH et al.** *The MFMU Cesarean Registry: factors affecting the success of trial of labor after previous cesarean delivery.* Am J Obstet Gynecol, 2005 ; 193 : 1016-1023.
60. **Seoud M, Nassar A, Usta I, Melhem Z, Kazma A, Khalil A**. *Impact of advance maternal age on pregnancy outcome*. Am J Perinatol, 2002; 19 : 1-7.
61. **Molloy BG, Sheil O, Duignan NM**. *Delivery after cesarean section: review of 2,176 consecutive cases.* Br Med J, 1987; 294: 1645-7.
62. **Ollendorff DA, Goldberg JM, Minogue JR, Socol ML.** *Vaginal birth after cesarean section for arrest of labor: is success determined by maximum cervical dilatation during the prior labor?* Am J Obstet Gynecol, 1988; 159: 636-9.

63. **Flamm BL, Goings JR.** *Vaginal birth after cesarean section: is suspected fetal macrosomia a contraindication?* Obstet Gynecol.1989; 74: 694-7.

64. **Olshan AF.** *Comparison of trial of labor with an elective second cesarean section.* N Engl J Med 1996; 335: 689-95.

65. **Roger V, Barret J, Bossart H, Lewin D, Renaud R**. *Traité d'obstétrique : la grossesse pathologique dystocique.* tome II, Masson, Paris.1983.

66. **Merger R, Levy J, Melchior J.** *Précis d'obstétrique.* 6th edition. Paris : Masson.2001.

67. **Mehats C, Schmitz T, Marcellin L, Breuiller-Fouche M.** *Biochemistry of premature rupture of fetal membranes.* GynecolObstet Fert.2001; 39: 365-69.

68. **Dyack C, Hughes PF, Simbakalia J.** *Vaginal delivery in the grand multipara following previous lower segment cesarian section.* J Obstet Gynaecol Res 1997; 23, 2: 219-222.

69. **Riethmuller D, Schaal JP.** *Preservation of membranes before large extraction of a second twin in transverse presentation.* La lettre du gynécilogue N°296 novembre 2004.

70. **Bensaid F, Filali A, Moussaoui DR, Bezad R, Chraibi C, El Fihri S, Alaoui T.** *Delivery of scar uteri at the C*
Rabat, Morocco, about 200 cases. Rev Fr Gynécol Obstet 1996**;** 91, 5: 217-22.

71. **Weinstein D, Benshushan A, T Anas V, Zilberstein R, Rojansky N.** *Predictive score for vaginal birth after cesarean section.* Am J Obstet Gynecol 1996; 174: 192-8.

72. **Kugler E, ShohamVardi I, Burstien E, Mazor M, Hershkovitz R.** *The safety of a trial of labor after cesarean section in a large multiparous population.* Arch Gynecol Obstet, 2008; 277: 339-44.

73. **Weinstein D, Benshushan A, Ezra Y, Rojansky N.** *Vaginal birth after cesarean section: current opinion.* Int. J. Gynecol. Obstet.1996; 53: 1-10.

74. **Benzineb M, Bellasfar B, Bouguerra MT, Amri R.** *Accouchement par voie basse après césarienne*. A propos de 173 épreuves.1998.

75. **Zwart JJ, Richters JM, Ory F, De Vries JI, Bloemenkamp KW, Van Roosmalen J.** *Uterine rupture in The Netherlands: a nationwide population-based cohort study.* BJOG, 2009; 116(8):1069-78.

76. **Al- Zirqi L, Stray-Pedersen B, Forsen L, Vangen S.** *Uterine rupture after previous caesarean section.* BJOG.2010; 117:809-20.

77. **Nabhan AF**. *Long term outcomes of two different surgical techniques for cesarean*, Intgynecol. Obstet .2007; sept. p 27.

78. **Aisien AO, Oronsaye AU.** *Vaginal birth after one previous caesarean section in a tertiary institution in Nigeria.* J Obstet Gynecol 2004; 24 (8): 886-890.

79. **Bais JM, Van Der Borden DMR, Pel M, Bonsel GJ, Eskes M, Van Der Slinke HJW et al.** *Vaginal birth after caesarean section in a population with low overall caesarean rate*. Eur. J Obstet Gynecol Reprod Biol 2001; 96: 158-162.

80. **Gyamfi C, Juhasz G, Gyamfi P, Stone JL**. Increased success of trial of labor after previous vaginal birth after cesarean. *Obstet Gynecol*.2004; 104:715-9.

81. **Hannah ME, Hannah WJ, Hewson SA**. *Planned Cesarean section versus planned vaginal birth for breech presentation at term: a randomized multicenter trial*. Lancet, 2000; vol. 356, p. 1375-83.

82. **Phelan JP, Ahn MO, Diaz F, Brar HS.** *Twice a Cesarean, always a Cesarean?* Obstet Gynecol 1989; vol. 73, p. 161-5.

83. **Mozurkewich L E, Hutton E.K.** *Elective repeat cesarean delivery versus trial of labor: A meta- analysis of the literature from 1989 to 1999*. Am. J Obstet Gynecol 2000;183 (5): 1187-1197.

84. **Maisonneuve AS, Haumonte JB, Carcopino X, Shojai R, Bretelle F, Chau C et al.** *Obstetrical outcome and risk of uterine rupture following a*

caesarean section before 32week. J Gynecol Obstet Biol Reprod, 2011; 40:334-9.

85. **Chauhan S, Magann E, Caroll CS, Barilleaux PS, Scardo JA, Martin JN.** *Mode of delivery for the morbidly obese with prior cesarean delivery: vaginal versus repeat cesarean section.* Am J Obstet Gynecol.2001;1S5:349-54.
86. **Ford AA, Bateman BT, Simpson LL.** *Vaginal birth after caesarean delivery in twin gestations: a large, nationwide sample of deliveries.* Am J. Obstet Gynecol 2006; 195 : 1138 - 1142.
87. **Kayem G, Raiffort C, Legardeur H, Gavard L, Mandelbort L, Girard G.** *Vaginal route acceptance criteria according to uterine scar characteristics.* J Gynecol Obstet Biol Reprod, 2012; 41:753-771.
88. **El Mansouri A.** *Accouchements sur uterus cicatriciel : A propos de 150 cas.* Rev. Fr Gynécol Obstét, 1994; 89 (12): 606-612.
89. **Abbassi H, Aboulfalah A, El Karroumi M, Bouhya S, Bekkay M.** *Delivery of scar uteri: can the uterine test be widened?* J. Gynecol. Obstet Biol Reprod1998; 27: 425-429.
90. **Roosmalen J.** *Vaginal birth after caesarean section in rural Tanzania.* Int J Gynecol Obstet, 1991; 34: 211-215.
91. **Rageth JC, Juzu C, Grossenbacher H.** Delivery after previous cesarean: A risk evaluation. Obstet. Gynecol.1999; 93: 332-337.
92. **Zine S, Abed A, Sfar E, Mouelhi T, Chelli H.** *Les ruptures utérines au cours du travail : A propos de 160 cas observés au center de maternité de Tunis.* Rev Fr gynécol Obstét 1995; 90 (3), 166-173.

Félix MOMAT KITENGE

Born on December 04, 1978 in Lubumbashi, Democratic Republic of Congo, Félix MOMAT KITENGE has held a Master's degree in Hautes Etudes de Stratégie et Défense at the Collège des Hautes Etudes de Stratégies et de Défense (CHESD) in Kinshasa since July 2019. In July 2017, he brilliantly defended an Agrégation de l'Enseignement Supérieur thesis in Medicine at the University of Lubumbashi, at the end of which he was awarded "LA PLUS GRANDE DISTICTION" with the Jury's Congratulations.

Félix MOMAT KITENGE holds a Master's degree in Emergency Medical Care Planning and Implementation from Yonsei University, South Korea (July 2013), and has been a specialist in Gynecology-Obstetrics at the University of Lubumbashi since July 2011, the same university that awarded him his Doctorate in Medicine in July 2004, after a brilliant primary and secondary education at Collège Imara Saint François des Sales in Lubumbashi, where he respectively obtained his primary school certificate (1992) and his state diploma in the Biology-Chemistry option (1998).

Félix MOMAT KITENGE is Associate Professor at the University of Lubumbashi in the Democratic Republic of Congo. He teaches at several other universities in the country (Université de Kalemie, Université de Kolwezi, Université Pédagogique du Congo, Institut Supérieur des Techniques Médicales de Lubumbashi, Institut Supérieur du Commerce de Lubumbashi, etc.).

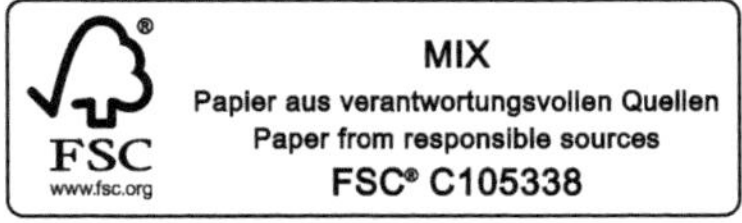

Printed by Books on Demand GmbH, Norderstedt / Germany